Tsuku Kihon

Dynamic Kumite Techniques of Shotokan Karate

2nd Edition

Luis Bernardo Mercado

authorHOUSE®

AuthorHouse™ LLC
1663 Liberty Drive
Bloomington, IN 47403
www.authorhouse.com
Phone: 1-800-839-8640

Published by AuthorHouse   06/24/2014

ISBN: 978-1-4772-8928-0 (sc)
ISBN: 978-1-4772-8927-3 (e)

Library of Congress Control Number: 2012921315

Contents

Appendix

Contributors

Front cover art, inside karate kihon and kata sketches, and author portrait, by Nobu Kaji, San Francisco.

Back cover art by Mike Thompson, Cloverdale, CA.

Samurai scene art by Egil Thompson, Cloverdale, CA.

I had the honor of contributing terms and definitions found in Chapter One of this book to sensei Steve McCann's excellent book, 'Karate Everyone, 2nd Edition.' Sensei McCann graciously gave permission for use of an edited version of those terms and definitions in this book.

Review and input by:

> Shojiro Sugiyama, JKA Chicago
>
> Jon Keeling, Silicon Valley Shotokan Karate
>
> Jose Novoa

In addition to the author, the following black belt instructors appear in pictures, thanks to all!

> Sensei Al McGaughey
>
> Sensei Harry Imamura
>
> Sensei Peter Rodriguez
>
> Sempai Cole Barber
>
> Sempai Lisa Cresta
>
> Sempai Kevin Little
>
> Sempai Ekapol Rojpiboonphun

Acknowledgments

Thank you to my family and friends, the most important people in my life.

I owe a great debt of gratitude to my long-time karate instructor, sensei Leroy Rodrigues, who is the most knowledgeable and talented martial arts practitioner with whom I have had the pleasure of training. Sensei Rodrigues is a generous teacher and mentor who opens many doors and opportunities to everyone who trains under him. He founded Shinkyu Shotokan Karate at the South San Francisco Parks & Recreation Department almost 40 years ago and continues to teach there. Sensei Rodrigues' system embodies principles from both the older style of Shorinji Ryu taught by the late Richard 'Biggie' Kim, and the newer derivative style of Shotokan karate taught to him by Chuck Okimura, which was founded by Gichin Funakoshi in the early 20th century.

I also want to thank two other wonderful instructors, sensei Mayer Parry, Buchido – my first Shotokan instructor, with whom I began martial arts training at San Francisco State University in 1981. And, sensei Al McGaughey, Pine Waves Karate Academy – my third karate instructor, with whom I continued martial arts studies in 1997. I have the honor of counting sensei McGaughey, along with sensei Harry Imamura, as partners at the Fremont Shotokan Karate dojo.

I wish to acknowledge the following exceptional people who positively impact all aspects of martial arts in the San Francisco Bay Area: Leroy Rodrigues, Clarence Lee, Sam Ahtye, Bernard Edwards, Jim Larkin, Steve McCann, Pete Rabbitt, Ric Sherrod, Joji Mercado, Dennis Clima, Joe Garcia, Wayne Pernell, Lisa Cresta, Sue Miller, Nobu Kaji, Harry Imamura, Alan McGaughey, Mike Thompson, Chester Chan, Jay Castellano, Henry Larkin, Jon Keeling, Rick Llewellyn, Marty Callahan, Dawn Flick, Peter Rodriguez, Anthony Corpuz, John Leggett, Stuart Sakai, and many others who are friends of the Fremont Shotokan Karate and Shinkyu Shotokan Karate dojos.

I also want to acknowledge the following masters, whose technical ability and karate proficiency are rarely achieved by any martial arts practitioner.

Hirokazu Kanazawa – Shotokan Karate International

Nobuaki Kanazawa – Shotokan Karate International

Steve Ubl – World Traditional Karate Organization

Richard Amos – World Traditional Karate Organization

Troy Price – Shuri-Te Bujutsu-Kai

Elmar Schmeisser – Shinkyu Shotokan Karate

Abe Quiane – Shotokan Karate

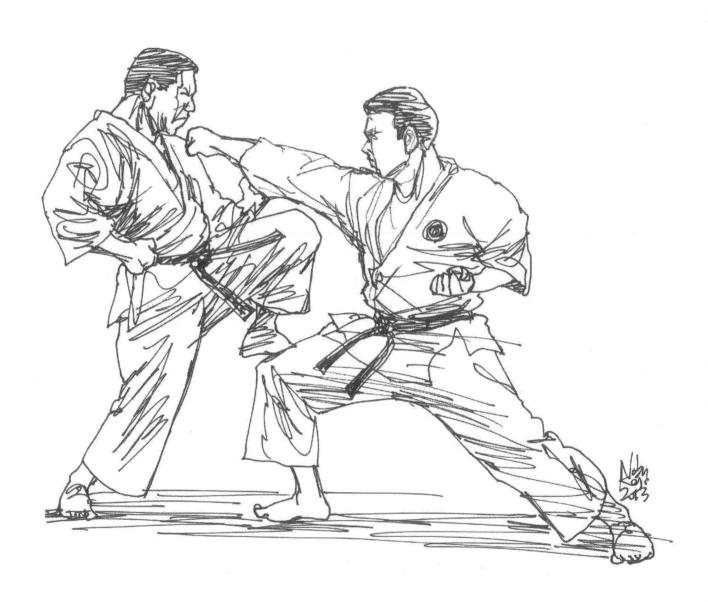

Chapter One
Introduction

This second edition of Tsuku Kihon is expanded to include several more exercises that will help practitioners improve their skills in this art form. Chapter 3 is for instructors to use as an introduction of Tsuku Kihon to beginners below brown belt. These exercises teach how to drop into an attack and end up in a complete front stance. Chapters 10 and 11 are meant for advanced students who have been training in Tsuku Kihon for about one year. Using the heavy bag and makiwara will sharpen skill at all levels and improve kime and distancing. Chapter 14 integrates sweeps into Tsuku Kihon combinations, which will raise kumite to a higher level of proficiency. Together, these additional drills will make for a more rounded martial arts practitioner, competitor, and improve self-defense capabilities.

Another great addition to this updated book is beautiful artwork by Nobu Kaji (tsuku kihon, kihon, and kata techniques), Egil Thompson (samurai scene drawings) and Mike Thompson (wood inlay artwork for back cover). All these original works of art give a sense of real action and martial arts spirit.

Tsuku Kihon is a phrase that I coined, which refers to advanced combat techniques used and taught by some Shotokan karate instructors. The idea behind Tsuku Kihon is that power and closing distance are greatly enhanced by propelling the body forward using dynamic karate principles. Sensei Leroy Rodrigues teaches these techniques at the Shinkyu Shotokan Karate dojo in South San Francisco, California. According to sensei Rodrigues, he learned them from sensei Chuck Okimura at his San Jose dojo sometime in the late 1970's.

A basic group of approximately 25 Tsuku Kihon techniques and combinations were developed by several Shotokan karate instructors in the middle part of the twentieth century. Sensei Rodrigues took them to a higher level in terms of execution and systemization.

After training under sensei Rodrigues for more than 25 years, I decided to expand and categorize the Tsuku Kihon in order to increase its applications and to create a formal structure for teaching them. After many months of trial and error, my efforts resulted in an additional 42 combinations and three methods by which Tsuku Kihon can be systematically taught to intermediate and advanced karate students.

Tsuku Kihon (tsuku means "push" in Japanese) should only be taught to brown and higher belts because lower-ranking students will not have the necessary karate foundation to understand and correctly execute them. Another way to look at this is that a student should have regularly trained for at least three years before learning Tsuku Kihon. Regular kihon ("basic" or "fundamentals" in Japanese) must first be understood and practiced by students for several years prior to being exposed to Tsuku Kihon.

Before we get into the actual techniques and how they work, let's first consider a few terms used in traditional martial arts. Many variables make up an effective martial art and, by extension, realistic self-defense techniques and mental attitude. Below is a partial list of terms that will serve to set the foundation to understand Shotokan karate principles.

Budo – The way of the warrior, or the way of martial arts. Term originally applied to the Japanese class known as Samurai. These men and women lived a life full of the constant threat of mortal combat. When one speaks of the way of the warrior in modern times, we refer to dedicating oneself to a code of honor, readiness, respect, humility, and an intense appreciation of life. A samurai's most important priority in life was honor, and he would commit suicide if he felt he had dishonored himself.

We don't expect martial artists to go to those lengths today, but we do place importance on budo basic virtues. Budo applies to everything we do, including our work, home life, social interactions, even driving. At work, for example, budo means that we do everything to the best of our ability and maintain the highest ethical standards. Therefore, work is not something into which we put just enough effort to get by and receive a paycheck. Even the most monotonous and lowly work must be done with pride and care. Training in the martial arts also requires that we strive to put in maximum effort and dedication at all times.

Choushi – Rhythm, especially related to performing techniques during katas or attacks against an opponent. Kata's are groups of self-defense techniques which follow predetermined patterns. When executed properly, katas are dynamic and interesting. When a kata is performed without proper rhythm, it is like playing music without meter.

Do – The "way" of…for example, Ken-do, Ju-do, Karate-do, Aiki-do, Bu-do. This term generally means to live one's life according to the principles and morals of a martial arts warrior. That is to say: treating people with respect, behaving in an honorable manner, practicing the martial arts diligently, seeking justice and truth, and being honest and pure of intention. Therefore, "Do" does not merely apply to the way one trains in karate but to the way we behave in every aspect of our lives. In other words, "Do" does not begin and end at the dojo entrance; it permeates every aspect of our lives.

Fudoshin – Immovable mind, imperturbability of mind in times of emergency, strong will. Some people have innate Fudoshin, while others must develop it over time, if at all. Most martial arts help to develop Fudoshin through discipline, commitment and training. Another way of looking at this is as the will to overcome any obstacle or adversity.

Go No Sen – Block, shift or retreat when an opponent attacks, then counter-attack. This mode of defense is the most common reaction to an attack because our natural instinct is to avoid being hit.

Hara – Concept of the "center"; the center of existence, the abdominal region, etc. Kime ("power," "intent," "commitment," "decisiveness," in Japanese) is said to originate from just below the navel when using proper karate techniques and having a proper attitude. When executing techniques, the hara is what unites the actions of the body and mind in order to achieve maximum impact. A strong hara also helps make the person more resistant to blows against the body.

Hyoshi – Timing. This term is similar to Choushi or rhythm but relates mainly to kumite ("sparring" in Japanese). As with rhythm, correct timing is important and can be the difference between winning and losing a battle. Timing is connected to accuracy because executing a good technique requires that it land in the right place at the right time.

Karate Ni Sente Nashi – "There is no first strike (nor offensive) in Karate." This is the first precept of karate-do. A martial artist should never be the one to start a conflict or throw the first punch. That is why it is said that most karate katas begin with a defensive technique.

Sensei Gichin Funakoshi also said "Karate begins and ends with respect." Having this attitude reduces the chance of getting into conflicts and needing to use violence. This precept is sometimes hard to follow, especially if someone attacks you.

There is a contradictory but equally valid rule which states that "If someone is going to attack you, hit them first and hit them hard." One can imagine that, after reaching a very high level in martial arts, one will almost never be in a situation that can't be settled peacefully so violence is averted altogether. Or, if someone does attack, we have already sensed a threat and kept enough distance to enable evasion or self-defense maneuvers.

Kiai – From "ki" and "ai" which is a contraction of the Japanese verb "awasu," i.e. "to unite," or, literally "spirit meeting," used in Bujutsu to coordinate and mobilize energy, used at the point of impact when executing a technique. Shouting the kiai increases power by uniting technique, strength, will power, spirit and focus at the moment of impact.

The kiai is itself considered a unique technique that must be developed and perfected. The kiai also helps clear the mind and eliminate fear during actual combat. It is said that an old master in Japan could knock birds off tree branches with his kiai alone. In fact, a strong and sharp kiai can end a fight because the attacker may think you are crazy or sense your power and decide that you are not someone he should mess with.

Kiai must be executed at the exact moment of impact in order for it to have maximum effectiveness. One additional benefit to kiai is that it forces air out of the lungs, which is correct for most offensive and defensive techniques. The act of expelling air, kime, proper technique, and kiai working together make karate very powerful indeed and an effective form of self-defense.

Kihon – basic karate techniques and stances.

Kime – focus and intensity when executing a technique. Martial arts without kime is merely posing or dancing. Every technique we execute must have an appropriate level of kime for effective application. Even gentle or slow moves have kime that is appropriate to that move. Kime is the coming together of intent, focus, technique, and spirit in order to achieve maximum power at the moment of impact.

Kime is said to originate from the hara, the center of the human body and crucible of courage and will. Spirit, in the context of martial arts, is not the same as religious or supernatural spirit. Spirit, in the context of kime can be described as an intense enthusiasm and will to achieve a task. In practical terms, the martial artist develops kime through practice and proper principles when executing techniques. One important element in developing good kime is to perform all moves with the tail bone tucked in and keeping the back straight. This proper posture aligns the body and maximizes balance, both of which are critical to proper execution of karate moves.

Ma Ai – The ability to accurately judge the distance between two competitors in kumite. Understanding distance, as well as timing and rhythm, is important in martial arts. By mastering all three, we increase the chance of being victorious in combat. Ma ai is more of a feeling or intuition than an actual conscious calculation and is developed over time with proper training. Ma ai can be thought of as similar to a basketball player trying to make a shot without needing to use a measuring tape to figure out how far he needs to shoot the ball. Over time, the practitioner gets a feel for distance without even thinking about it.

Mushin – Absence of mind; acting subconsciously; reacting without the use of conscious thought. This refers to the ability to react to an attack without thought or delay. Mushin is analogous to a child learning how to walk and eventually being able to do it without giving it any thought. Another way to look at this is as developing muscle memory. The body simply reacts properly because that is how years of training have conditioned it. This kind of thing happens in its own time and can't be forced or hurried; only proper training and dedication can bring it about.

Sen No Sen – Confidence in fighting can often lead to beating an opponent to the punch, even though he initiated his attack first. This form of dealing with an attack is very advanced. It also takes a lot of courage because one must focus more on landing one's counter strike than on the threat of the opponent's strike, which one knows was launched before ours. When it works, the defender is at a great disadvantage initially but still is victorious because of his courage, impeccable technique, and perfect timing.

Sensei – Teacher. The senior instructor of the dojo ("training hall" in Japanese), typically 4th dan (black belt level or degree) or higher. The sensei is more than just an instructor; he is also a mentor and a reservoir of years of experience and knowledge. Students must appreciate the years of dedication and effort that a person has invested to reach the level of sensei.

At the same time, the sensei is not super human or perfect. In fact, the sensei is a student as well because every time he steps on the dojo floor to teach he must be open to learning more about the things he teaches. A sensei can be thought of as the most senior student in the class. A sensei deserves respect and his instructions must be followed with dedication and focus.

Very few people will have the dedication and skill to reach the level of sensei. But it should be the goal of every serious student to reach that level and someday impart their knowledge to a new generation of students. As sensei's, we sincerely hope that our students will reach greater levels of skill and dedication than we have.

Zanshin – Readiness during combat or training. Refers to being ready to defend or attack at any point in time during combat. In Kumite, Zanshin refers to having your guard up at every instant while engaging the opponent. Zanshin is not only having the body in a ready position, it is also an attitude of always being ready to defend or attack. Some people have natural ability in the martial arts and Zanshin comes easy for them. But for most of us it takes time, dedication and practice to develop this state of awareness and focus.

Understanding and practicing the above concepts is essential to advanced martial arts training and self-defense applications.

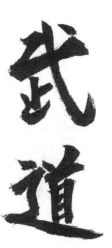

武道

Budo

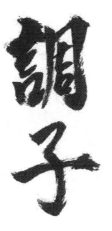

調子

Choushi

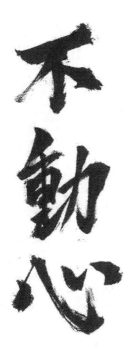

不動心

Fudoshin

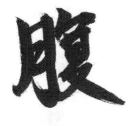

腹

Hara

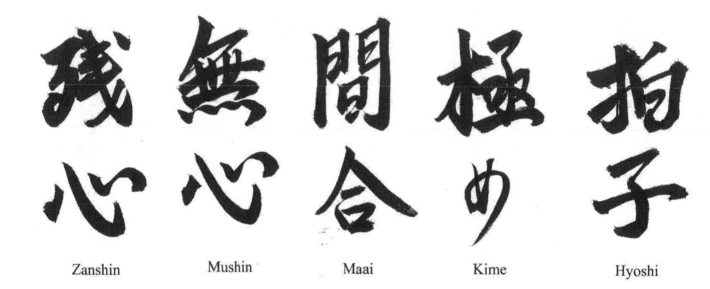

残心　無心　間合　極め　拘子

Zanshin　Mushin　Maai　Kime　Hyoshi

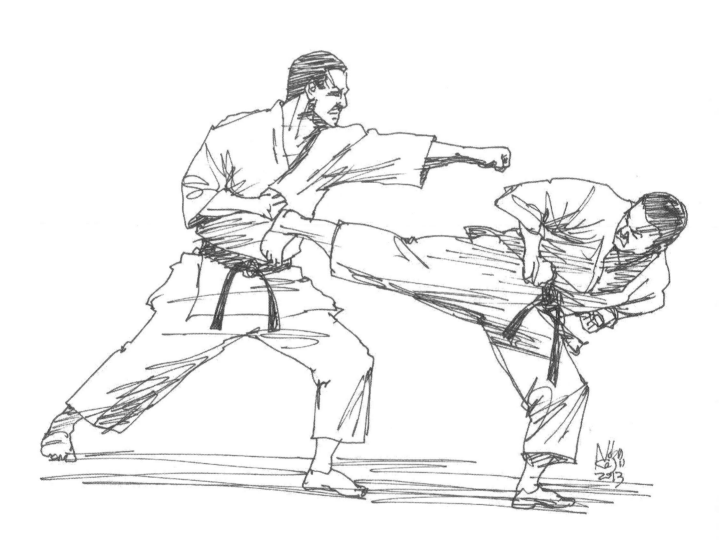

Chapter Two
Basic Karate Concepts

Kamae, as defined here and in its most basic form, is a natural fighting stance that is slightly shorter than zenkutso dachi and with the rear leg a bit more compressed. The front hand is at chin level, palm up, with the index and middle knuckles directed at the opponent's nose. The other hand is at solar plexus level, palm up, with the index and middle knuckles directed at the opponent's sternum. All Tsuku Kihon starts and ends in kamae.

Stance at the point of impact is a basic Shotokan zenkutsu dachi (front stance). In techniques where the rear foot steps forward, movements are executed in quick, snapping motions with the feet staying close to the ground.

Certain techniques and combinations require a reset step to get back to kamae. The reset step is typically done with the rear foot taking a small step forward and then the front foot taking a small step forward. Not all Tsuku Kihon combinations require a reset step, as will be demonstrated in the chapters to follow.

Keys to effective Tsuku Kihon execution:

> When the strike is a lunge or reverse punch, the hip is at a right angle to the front leg. The hip is at 135 degrees to the front leg for jabs, or another way to look at it is that the hip is at 45 degrees to the target. The angled position for a jab is equivalent to a defensive stance where the body is skewed so as to present a smaller target.
> Maximum power is achieved by propelling the body forward so that most of the body's mass is behind a strike at the moment of impact. As we may all know, speed plus mass equals power, so the quicker that forward motion is performed, the more power that is delivered to the target at the moment of impact.
> The rear leg is bent and compressed like a coiled spring. When a forward technique is executed, the rear leg initiates forward motion by exploding into a nearly straight position. This is analogous to a coiled spring releasing stored energy.
> With any striking technique, the body needs to compress at the point of impact. The tension begins in the stomach muscles below the navel, and ends with tightening various extremities so that a large part of the body becomes one solid unit for a fraction of a second. The tailbone also tucks in, adding stability and proper posture throughout most of the motion and at the point of impact. Immediately after striking the target, the body must relax to be ready for the next move.
> The pull-back hand must be withdrawn quickly to the hip or used to block an opponent's strike. When practicing kihon, the pull-back hand always retreats to the hip. In combat situations the pull-back hand can be used to block or to grab an incoming leg or arm.
> When stepping forward, sideways, or back, knees are bent so as to keep body height the same. When attacking, height will actually shorten because of body compression.
> In techniques where the front foot moves forward, the feeling should be of one dropping into the

target.

- ➤ The front foot should point towards the opponent's center and remain aligned that way when moving in any direction. The movement grid is a semi-circle around the opponent's front with our body pointing like an arrow towards his center.

- ➤ The legs should not cross over each other at any time, and our body mass is positioned slightly in front of the center of our body.

- ➤ We should exhale, usually, when attacking and, if possible, inhale between combinations. Our lungs should never be completely emptied.

- ➤ Distance and technique type change depending on the type of rear leg forward step. For example, when the rear foot takes a quarter-step forward and the lead hand punches, that is a jab. However, when the rear foot takes a full step forward and the lead hand punches, that is a reverse punch.

- ➤ The first technique can be a feint or distraction. In other words, a technique is not only used with the intent to strike, it can also be used as a fake in order to disguise what's coming up next.

- ➤ Rhythm and timing should be varied so as to be unpredictable.

- ➤ In sparring and pre-arranged training, attack and defense must be intense and realistic but without injuring the opponent. Therefore, the focal point of a technique at the point of impact should be just on the surface of the target… not through the target, as it would be during a real fight.

- ➤ Footwork rhythm depends on the combination being executed and how the opponent moves. Varying rhythm will make it harder for the opponent to predict when an attack is coming.

In the followings pages, sempai Lisa Cresta demonstrates step-by-step execution of a few relevant Shotokan basics. Some pages also include drawings of foot positions and step movements. Distance depicted in the diagrams is relative to the height of a person and how deep one wishes to do a stance. The depth of a stance may also depend on the distance to an opponent. Note that in the later drawings with more detail, the numbers depicted are in inches.

Front Stance (Zenkutsu Dachi)

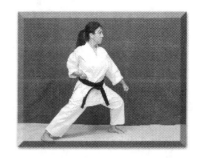

Ready Stance (Kamae)

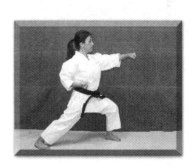

Reverse Punch (Gyaku Zuki)

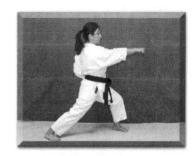

Lunge Punch (Oi Zuki)

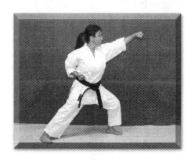

Jab (Kizami Zuki)

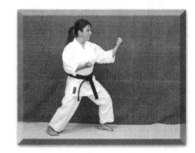

Ready Stance (Kamae)

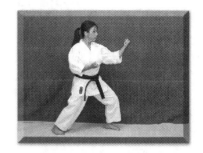

Kizami Gyaku Zuki Position A

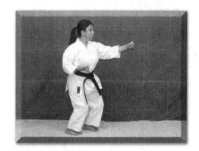

Kizami Gyaku Zuki Position B

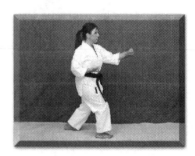

Kizami Gyaku Zuki Position C

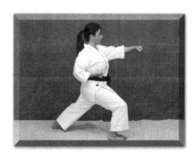

> Reverse punch with the front hand,
  taking a full step into front stance.

Tsuku Kihon Principles 3

Ready Stance (Kamae)

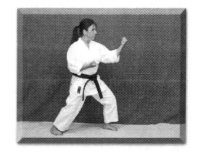

Rear Foot Half Step Forward

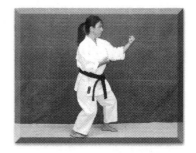

Rear Foot Half Step Back to Kamae

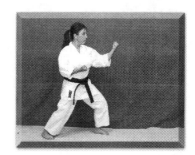

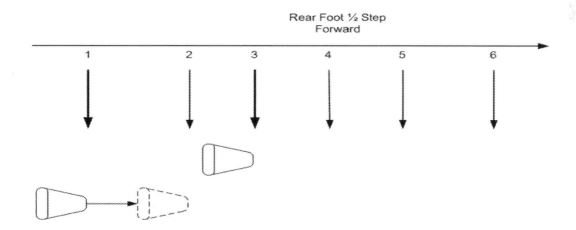

Rear Foot ½ Step
Forward

1   2   3   4   5   6

Tʂᴜᴋᴜ Kɪʜᴏɴ Pʀɪɴᴄɪᴘʟᴇꜱ 4

Ready Stance (Kamae)

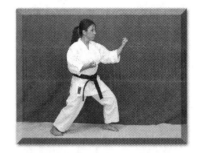

Front Foot Quarter Step Forward

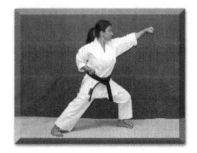

Front Foot Quarter Step Back to Kamae

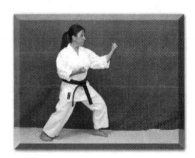

Front Foot ¼ Step
Forward

| 1 | 2 | 3 | 4 | 5 | 6 |

Tsuku Kihon Principles 5

Ready Stance (Kamae)

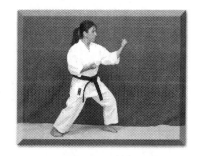

Front Foot Full Step Forward
 to Front Stance

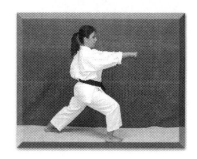

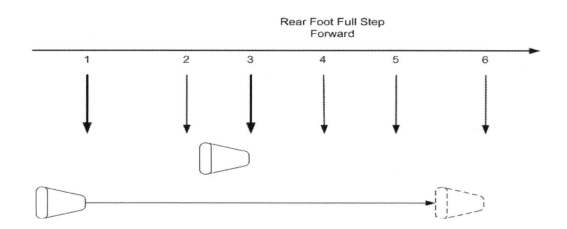

Tsuku Kihon Principles 6

Ready Stance (Kamae)

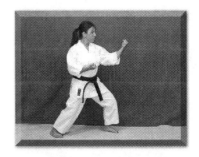

Rear Foot, Foot Replacement

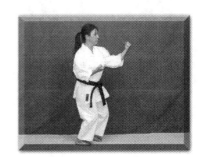

Foot Replacement Rear
Foot Forward

2 3 4 5 6

Ready Stance (Kamae)

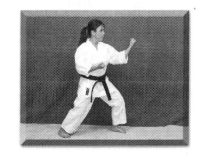

Front Snap Kick Chamber
(Mae Geri)

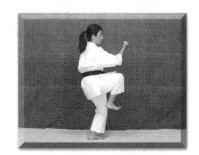

Front Snap Kick Extended

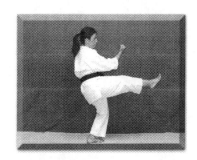

Front Snap Kick Chamber

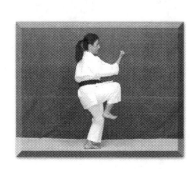

Ready Stance

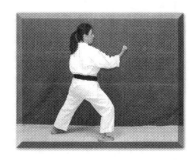

Ready Stance (Kamae)

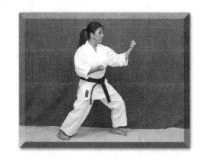

Round House Kick Chamber
(Mawashi Geri)

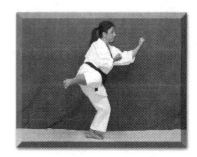

Round House Kick Extended

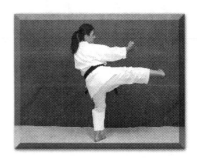

Round House Kick Chamber

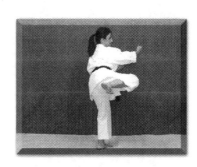

Ready Stance

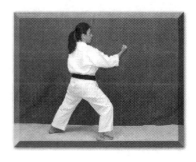

Ready Cat Stance (Nekoashi Dachi)

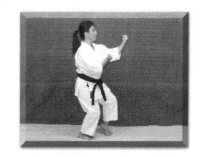

Front Leg Snap Kick Chamber
(Kizami Mae Geri)

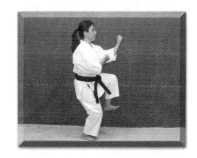

Front Leg Snap Kick Extended

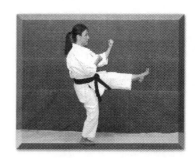

Front Leg Snap Kick Chamber

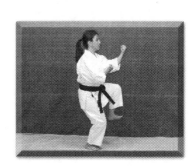

Ready Cat Stance

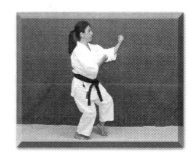

Ready Stance (Kamae)

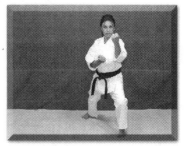

Side Thrust Kick Chamber
(Yoko Geri Keikome)

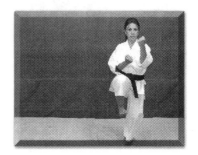

Side Thrust Kick Extended

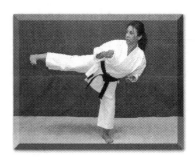

Side Thrust Kick Chamber

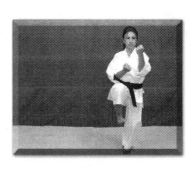

Ready Stance

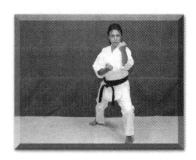

Ready Stance (Kamae)

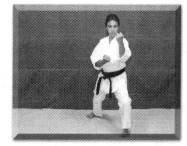

Side Snap Kick Chamber
(Yoko Geri Keage)

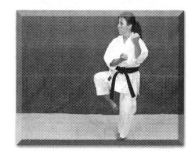

Side Snap Kick Extended

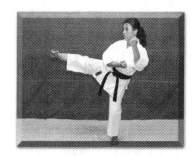

Side Snap Kick Chamber

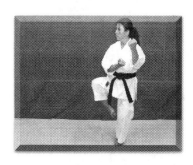

Ready Stance

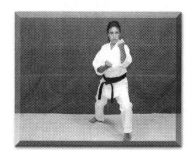

Front Stance - Zenkutsu Dachi

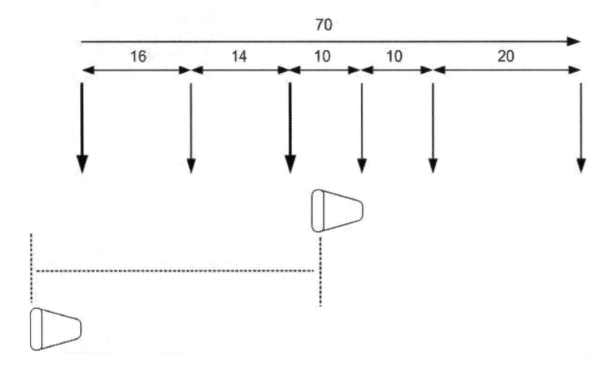

Fighting Stance - Kamae

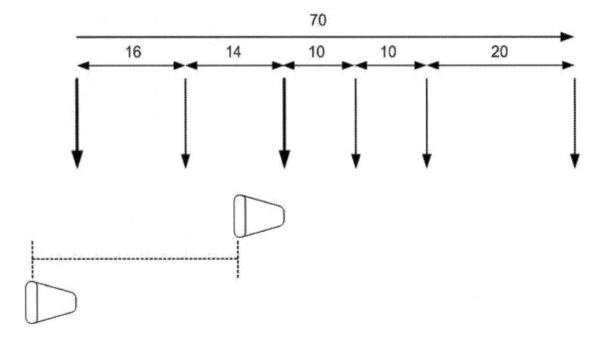

Front Foot ¼ Step Forward

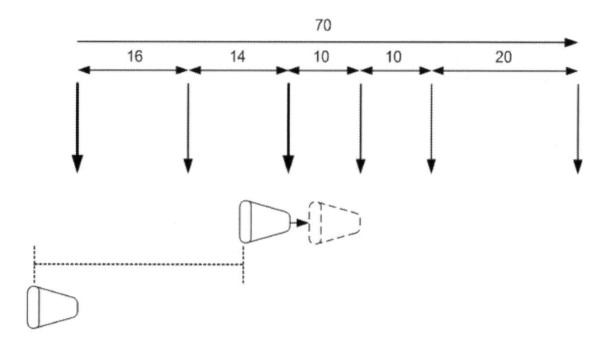

Rear Foot ½ Step Forward

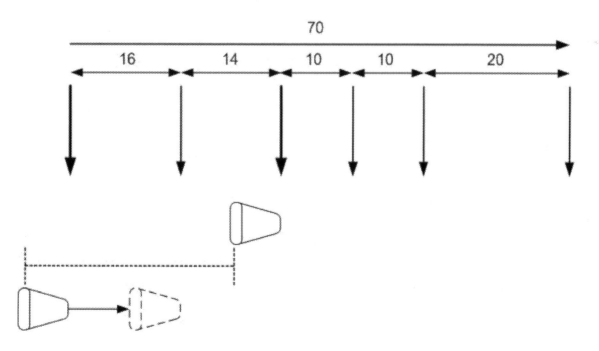

Front Foot ¼ Step Forward and Reset to Kamae

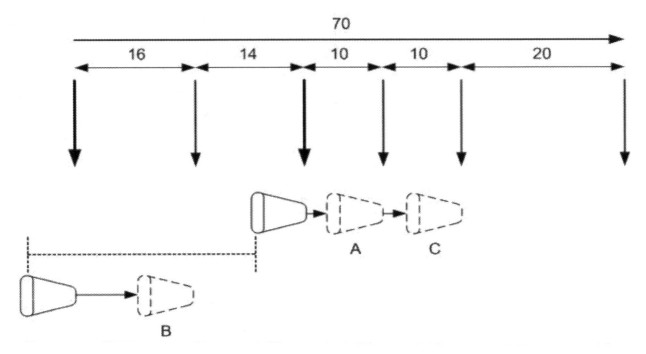

Rear Foot ½ Step Forward and Reset to Kamae

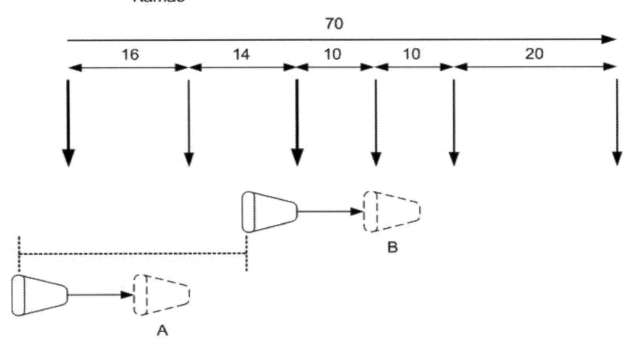

Rear Foot Full Step Forward to Zenkutsu Dachi

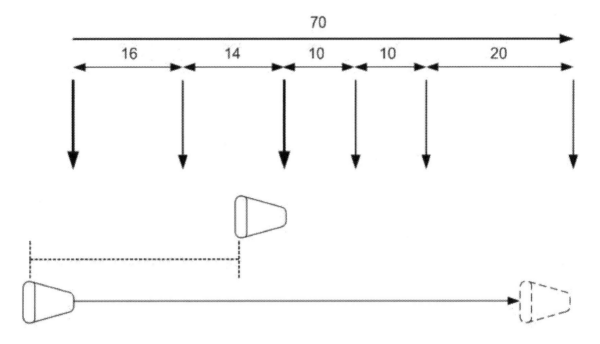

Rear Foot Forward Foot Replacement

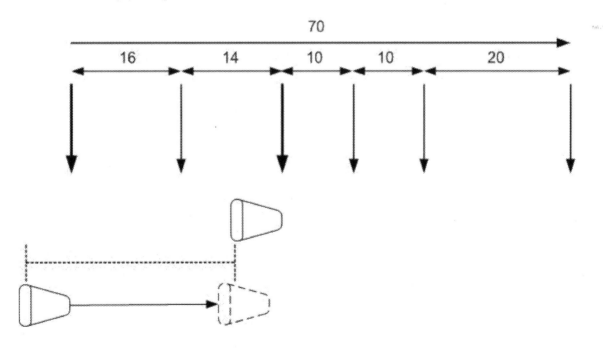

Rear Foot Full Step Forward to Zenkutsu Dachi and Reset to Kamai

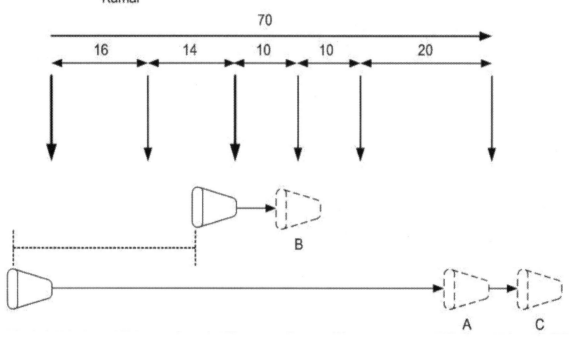

Rear Foot Forward Foot Replacement and Reset To Kamae

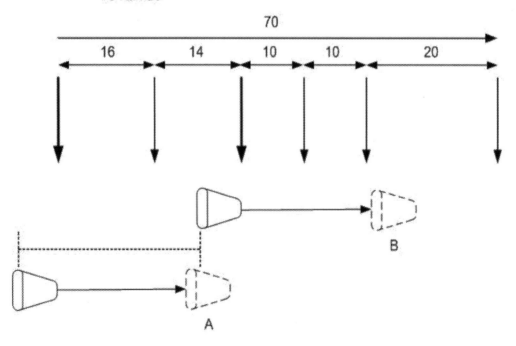

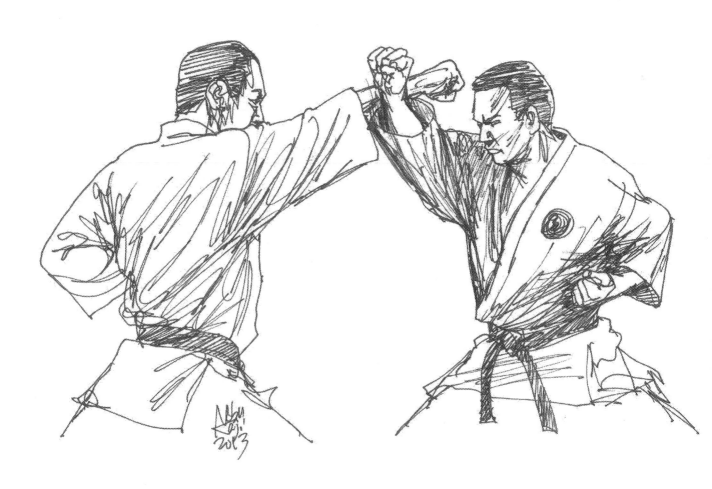

Chapter Three
Pre-Tsuku Kihon Drills

Prior to learning Tsuku Kihon techniques, we first must understand and practice several essential concepts intended to build up kime and dropping forward when attacking. Moreover, these building blocks are a practical application of Shotokan kihon for real combat and therefore lead us into Tsuku Kihon. These exercises can be taught to students just starting to learn karate.

Please note that not all drills listed below are pictured.

a. Natural stance, left arm in punch position, step forward with right foot lunge punch to front stance, step back to natural stance leaving right arm in punch position. Step forward with left foot lunge punch to front stance, step back to natural stance leaving left arm in punch position. Repeat 10 times.

b. Natural stance, left arm in punch position, step forward with left foot reverse punch to front stance, step back to natural stance leaving right arm in punch position. Step forward with right foot reverse punch to front stance, step back to natural stance leaving left arm in punch position. Repeat 10 times.

c. Natural stance, left arm in punch position, step forward with right foot lunge punch to front stance, then reverse punch, step back to natural stance leaving left arm in punch position. Repeat 10 times.

d. Natural stance, right arm in punch position, step forward with left foot lunge punch to front stance, then reverse punch, step back to natural stance leaving right arm in punch position. Repeat 10 times.

e. Natural stance, arms in square guard position, left foot front snap kick to front stance, step back to natural stance with arms in square guard position. Right foot front snap kick to front stance, step back to natural stance with arms in square guard position. Repeat 10 times.

f. Natural stance, arms in square guard position, left foot front snap kick, lunge punch to front stance, step back to natural stance with arms in square guard position. Right foot snap kick, lunge punch to front stance, step back to natural stance with arms in square guard position. Repeat 10 times.

g. Natural stance, left arm in punch position, right foot front snap kick lunge punch to front stance, step back to natural stance leaving right arm in punch position. Left foot front snap kick lunge punch to front stance, step back to natural stance leaving left arm in punch position. Repeat 10 times.

h. Natural stance, left arm in punch position, left foot front snap kick reverse punch to front stance, step back to natural stance leaving right arm in punch position. Right foot front snap kick reverse punch to front stance, step back to natural stance leaving left arm in punch position. Repeat 10 times.

i. Natural stance, left arm in punch position, right foot front snap kick lunge punch to front stance, then reverse punch, step back to natural stance leaving left arm in punch position. Repeat 10 times.

j. Natural stance, right arm in punch position, left foot front snap kick lunge punch to front stance, then reverse punch, step back to natural stance leaving right arm in punch position. Repeat 10 times.

k. Natural stance, arms in square guard position, left foot round house kick to front stance, step back to natural stance with arms in squared guard position. Right foot round house kick to front stance, step back to natural stance with arms in square kamae position. Repeat 10 times.

l. Natural stance, arms in square guard position, left foot round house kick reverse punch to front stance, step back to natural stance with arms in squared guard position. Right foot round house kick reverse punch to front stance, step back to natural stance with arms in square guard position. Repeat 10 times.

Pre Tsuku Kihon A

1) Natural Stance

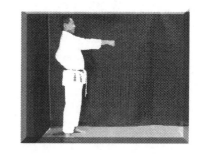

2) Drop Step Forward Lunge Punch
   to Front Stance

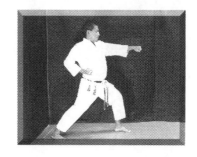

3) Front Leg Back to Natural Stance
   Leave Punch Hand Out

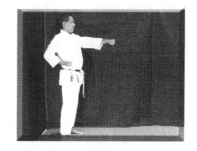

> Oi Zuki

Pre Tsuku Kihon B

1) Natural Stance

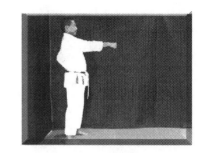

2) Drop Step Forward Reverse Punch
   to Front Stance

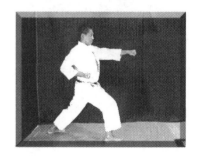

3) Front Leg Back to Natural Stance
   Leave Punch Hand Out

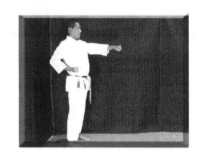

> Gyaku Zuki

Pre Tsuku Kihon C

1) Natural Stance

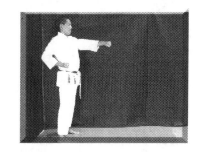

2) Drop Step Forward Lunch Punch
   to Front Stance

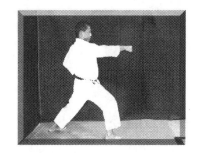

3) Reverse Punch

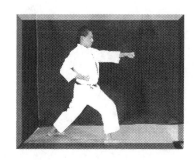

4) Step Back to Natural Stance,
   Leave Punch Hand Out

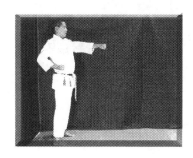

> Oi Zuki, Gyaku Zuki

Pre Tsuku Kihon F

1) Natural Guard Stance

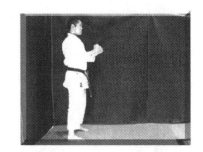

2) Execute Front Snap Kick While
   Dropping Forward

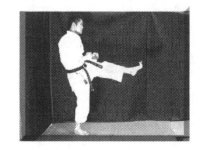

3) Drop Forward Lunch Punch
   to Front Stance

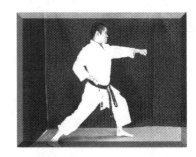

4) Step Back to Natural Guard Stance

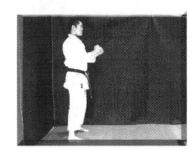

> Mae Geri, Oi Zuki

Pre Tsuku Kihon H

1) Natural Stance

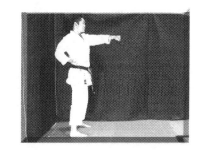

2) Execute Front Snap Kick While
   Dropping Forward

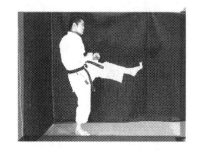

3) Drop Forward Reverse Punch
   to Front Stance

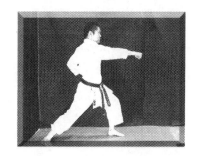

4) Step Back to Natural Stance, Leave
   Punch Hand Out

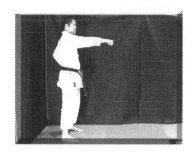

> Mae Geri, Gyaku Zuki

Pre Tsuku Kihon L

1) Natural Guard Stance

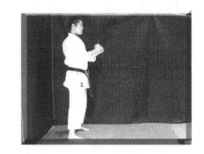

2) Execute Round House Kick
   While Dropping Forward

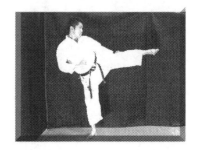

3) Drop Forward Reverse Punch
   to Front Stance

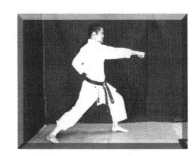

4) Step Back to Natural Guard Stance

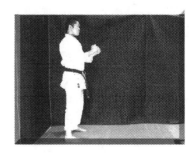

> Mawashi Geri, Gyaku Zuki

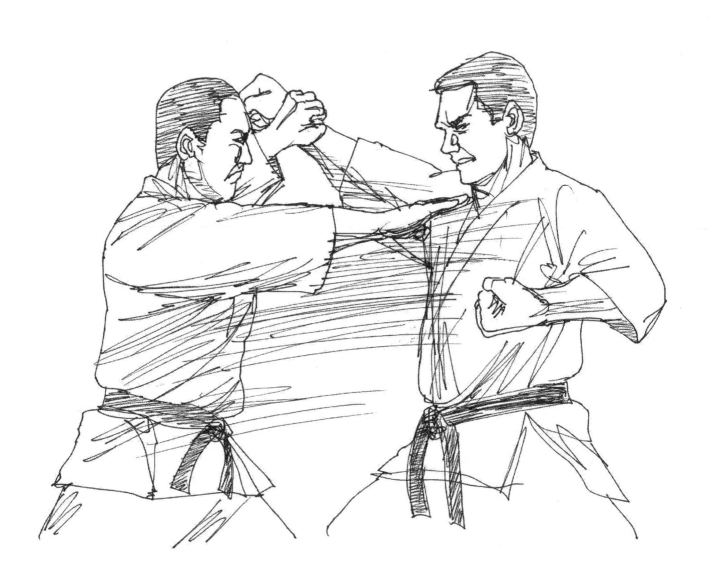

Chapter Four
Single Techniques

Tsuku Kihon is introduced with single techniques, which are its foundation, and should be thoroughly understood prior to linking them together to form the combinations that will follow in later chapters. These twelve basics are, essentially, the alphabet of Tsuku Kihon. Please note that picture sets in Chapters Three, Four, Five, Six and Eight are numbered according to the "Sequential" series order, which is listed in Chapter Thirteen.

1) kamae, front foot ¼ step forward jab, front foot back, kamae **(kizami zuki)***
2) kamae, front foot ¼ step forward jab, rear foot ½ step forward, front foot ¼ step forward, kamae **(kizami zuki)***
3) kamae, rear foot ½ step forward jab, rear foot ½ step back, kamae **(kizami zuki)***
4) kamae, rear foot ½ step forward jab, front foot ½ step forward, kamae **(kizami zuki)***
5) kamae, front foot ¼ step forward reverse punch, front foot back, kamae **(gyaku zuki)***
6) kamae, front foot ¼ step forward reverse punch, rear foot ½ step forward, front foot ¼ step forward, kamae **(gyaku zuki)***
7) kamae, front foot ¼ step forward reverse punch, rear foot full step forward, kamae **(oi gyaku zuki)***
8) kamae, front foot ¼ step forward back fist to full front stance, front foot back, kamae **(kizami uraken uchi)**
9) kamae, front foot ¼ step forward back fist to full front stance, rear foot ½ step forward, front foot ¼ step forward, kamae **(kizami uraken uchi)**
10) kamae, lunge punch to full front stance, rear foot ½ step forward, front foot ¼ step forward, kamae **(oi zuki)***
11) kamae, lunge back fist to full front stance, rear foot ½ step forward, front foot ¼ step forward, kamae **(oi uraken uchi)***
12) kamae, rear foot full step forward reverse punch with front hand, rear foot forward ½ step, front foot ¼ step forward, kamae **(kizami gyaku zuki)**

Tsuku Kihon 1

1) Ready Stance

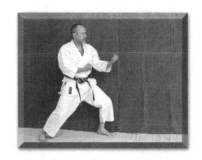

2) Front Leg 1/4 Step Forward Jab
   to Front Stance

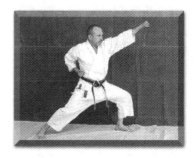

3) Front Leg Back to Ready Stance

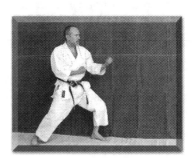

> Kizami Zuki

Tsuku Kihon 2

1) Ready Stance

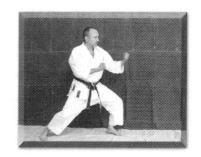

2) Front Foot 1/4 Step Forward Jab
   to Front Stance

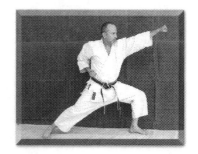

3) Rear Leg 1/2 Step Forward Transition

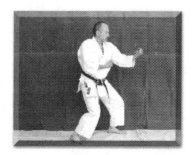

4) Front Leg Step Forward
   to Ready Stance

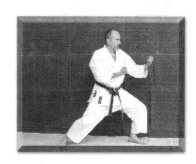

> Kizami Zuki

Tsuku Kihon 3

1) Ready Stance

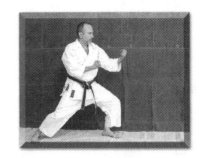

2) Rear Leg 1/2 Step Forward Jab

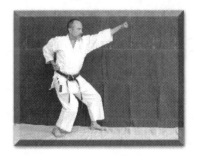

3) Rear Leg Step Back to Ready Stance

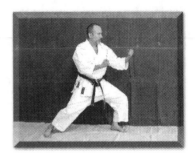

> Kizami Zuki

Tsuku Kihon 4

1) Ready Stance

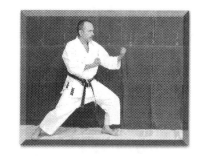

2) Rear Leg 1/2 Step Forward Jab

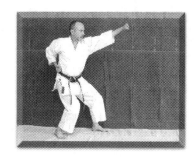

3) Front Leg Step Forward
   to Ready Stance

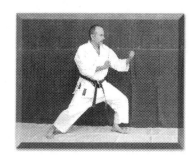

> Kizami Zuki

Tsuku Kihon 5

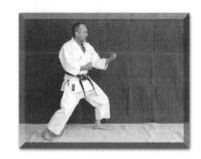

1) Ready Stance

2) Front Leg 1/4 Step Forward
   Reverse Punch to Front Stance

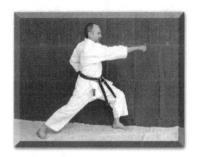

3) Front Leg Back to Ready Stance

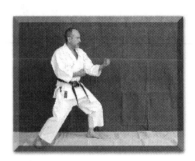

> Gyaku Zuki

Tsuku Kihon 6

1) Ready Stance

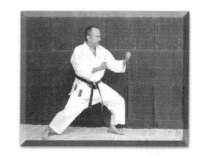

2) Front Foot 1/4 Step Forward
   Reverse Punch to Front Stance

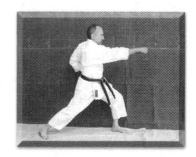

3) Rear Leg 1/2 Step Forward Transition

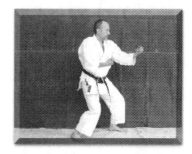

4) Front Leg Step Forward
   to Ready Stance

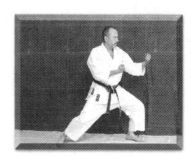

> Gyaku Zuki

1) Ready Stance

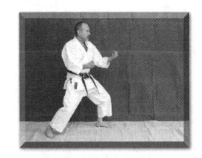

2) Front Foot 1/4 Step Forward
   Reverse Punch to Front Stance

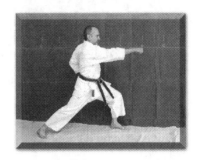

3) Full Step Forward to Ready Stance

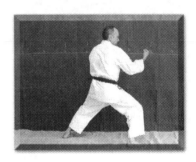

> Oi Gyaku Zuki

1) Ready Stance

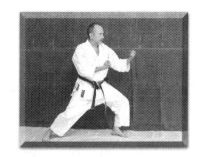

2) Front Leg 1/4 Step Forward
   Back Fist Strike

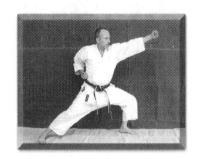

3) Front Leg Step Back to Ready Stance

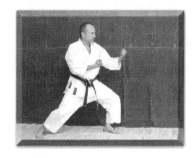

> Kizami Uraken Uchi

Tsuku Kihon 9

1) Ready Stance

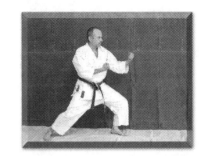

2) Front Foot 1/4 Step Forward
   Back Fist Strike

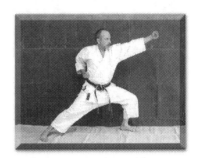

3) Rear Leg Forward 1/2 Step Transition

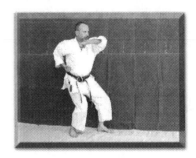

4) Front Leg Step Forward
   to Ready Stance

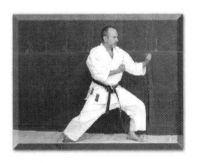

> Kizami Uraken Uchi

Tsuku Kihon 10

1) Ready Stance

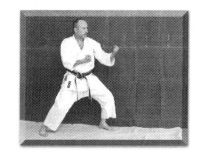

2) Lunge Punch to Front Stance

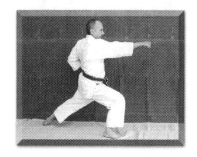

3) Rear Leg Forward 1/2 Step Transition

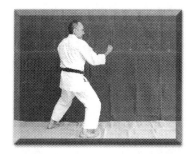

4) Front Leg Step Forward
   to Ready Stance

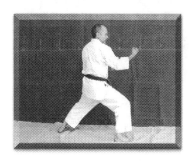

> Oi Zuki

1) Ready Stance

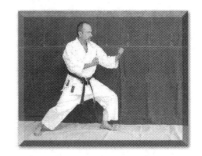

2) Step Transition Chamber
   Striking Hand

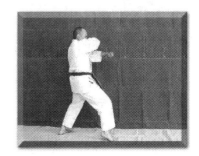

3) Back Fist Strike to Front Stance

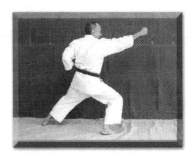

4) Rear Leg Forward 1/2 Step Transition

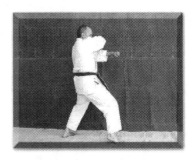

5) Front Leg Forward to Ready Stance

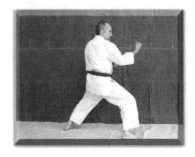

> Oi Uraken Uchi

1) Ready Stance

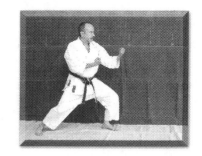

2) Rear Leg Full Step Forward
   Lead Hand Reverse Punch

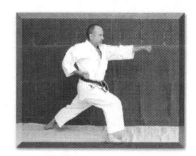

3) Rear Leg 1/2 Step Forward Transition

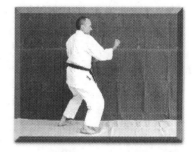

4) Front Leg Forward to Ready Stance

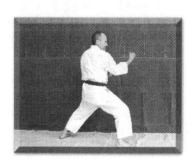

> Kizami Gyaku Zuki

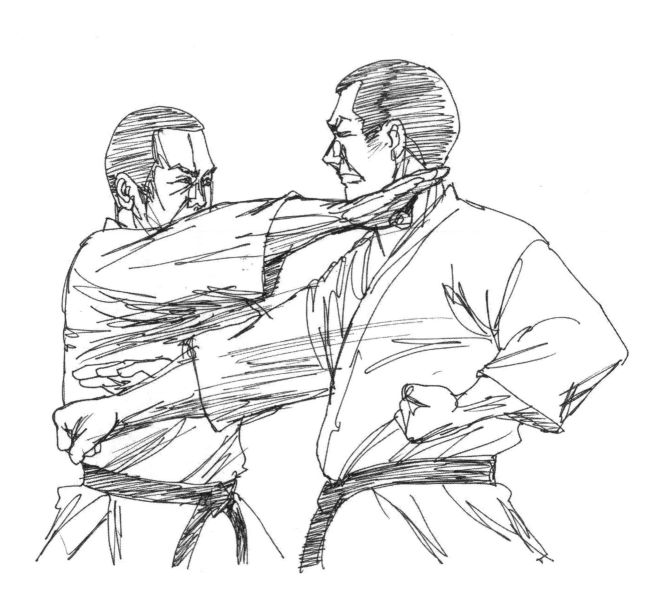

Chapter Five
Double-Technique Sequence

Two techniques executed one after the other is the most common application of Tsuku Kihon. In sparring or real combat, it is essential to finish off an opponent with one or two well-placed and powerful techniques. The idea is that if one faces a stronger attacker, he must be disabled or injured quickly because if the attacker is allowed to land a blow, he may do serious damage to the defender. Physical conditioning is another important element because an average person will become completely exhausted after only 15 to 30 seconds of real combat. Therefore, it is critical that an attacker be neutralized as soon as possible, preferably with just one or two devastating blows.

Please note that not all drills listed below are pictured.

o kamae, front foot ¼ step forward jab, rear foot ½ step forward, front foot ½ step forward reverse punch, rear foot ½ step forward, front foot ¼ step forward, kamae **(kizami zuki, gyaku zuki)***
o kamae, front foot ¼ step forward jab, reverse punch, bring front foot back, kamae **(kizami zuki, gyaku zuki)**
o kamae, rear foot ½ step forward jab, rear foot ½ step back reverse punch, kamae **(kizami zuki, gyaku zuki)**
o kamae, front foot ¼ step forward jab, lunge punch to full front stance, rear foot ½ step forward, front foot ¼ step forward, kamae **(kizami zuki, oi zuki)***
o kamae, rear foot ½ step forward jab, front foot ½ step forward reverse punch, rear foot ½ step forward, front foot ¼ step forward, kamae **(kizami zuki, gyaku zuki)**
o kamae, rear foot ½ step forward reverse punch, rear foot ½ step back jab, kamae **(gyaku zuki, kizami zuki)**
o kamae, front foot ¼ step forward reverse punch, same hand lunge back fist to full front stance, rear foot ½ step forward, front foot ¼ step forward, kamae **(gyaku zuki, oi uraken uchi)***
o kamae, front foot ¼ step forward reverse punch, rear leg front snap kick, rear foot ½ step forward, front foot ¼ step forward, kamae **(gyaku zuki, gyaku mae geri)***
o kamae, front foot ¼ step forward reverse punch, same hand lunge punch to full front stance, rear foot ½ step forward, front foot ¼ step forward, kamae **(gyaku zuki, oi zuki)**
o kamae, front foot ¼ step forward reverse punch, rear foot ½ step forward jab, front foot ¼ step forward, kamae **(gyaku zuki, kizami zuki)**
o kamae, front foot ¼ step forward reverse punch, rear foot full step forward reverse punch, rear foot ½ step forward, front foot ¼ step forward, kamae **(gyaku zuki, gyaku zuki)***
o kamae, lunge punch to full front stance, rear foot ½ step forward, front foot ¼ step forward same hand back fist, kamae **(oi zuki, oi uraken uchi)***
o kamae, lunge punch to full front stance, rear foot ½ step forward, front foot ¼ step forward reverse punch, rear foot ½ step forward, front foot ¼ step forward, kamae **(oi zuki, gyaku zuki)***
o kamae, lunge punch to full front stance, rear foot ½ step forward, front foot ¼ step forward same hand jab, rear foot ½ step forward, front foot ¼ step forward, kamae **(oi zuki, kizami zuki)***
o kamae, lunge punch to full front stance, rear foot ½ step forward, front leg front snap kick to full front stance, rear foot ½ step forward, front foot ¼ step forward, kamae **(oi zuki, kizami mae geri)**

- kamae, rear foot full step forward reverse punch with front hand, rear foot ½ step forward jab, front foot ¼ step forward, kamae **(kizami gyaku zuki, kizami zuki)**
- kamae, rear foot full step forward reverse punch with front hand, same hand lunge punch to full front stance, rear foot ½ step forward, front foot ¼ step forward, kamae **(kizami gyaku zuki, oi zuki)**
- kamae, rear leg round house kick, reverse punch to full front stance, rear foot ½ step forward, front foot ¼ step forward, kamae **(gyaku mawashi geri, gyaku zuki)***
- kamae, rear leg side thrust kick, lunge back fist to full front stance, rear foot ½ step forward, front foot ¼ step forward, kamae **(gyaku yoko geri, oi uraken uchi)***
- kamae, rear leg spinning back kick, reverse punch to full front stance, rear foot ½ step forward, front foot ¼ step forward, kamae **(uchiro geri, gyaku zuki)***
- kamae, rear leg front snap kick, lunge back fist to full front stance, rear foot ½ step forward, front foot ¼ step forward, kamae **(gyaku mae geri, oi uraken uchi)***
- kamae, rear leg front snap kick, lunge punch to full front stance, rear foot ½ step forward, front foot ¼ step forward, kamae **(gyaku mae geri, oi zuki)***
- kamae, front leg snap kick, same side jab to full front stance, front foot back, kamae **(kizami mae geri, kizami zuki)**

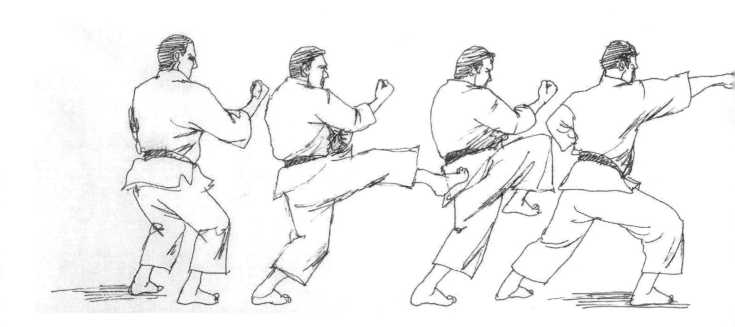

Tsuku Kihon 13

1) Ready Stance

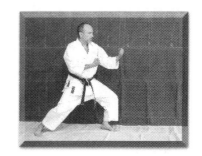

2) Front Foot 1/4 Step Forward Jab
to Front Stance

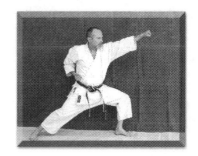

3) Reverse Punch

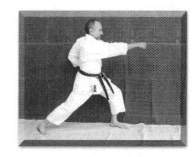

4) Front Leg Back to Ready Stance

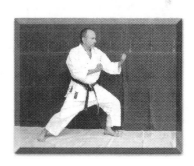

> Kizami Zuki, Gyaku Zuki

1) Ready Stance

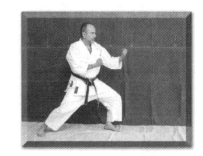

2) Rear Foot 1/2 Step Forward Jab

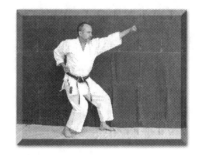

3) Rear Foot Step Back to Front Stance
   Reverse Punch

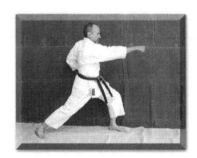

4) Rear Foot Step Forward
   to Ready Stance

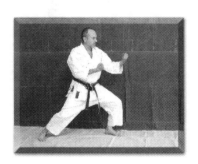

> Kizami Zuki, Gyaku Zuki

1) Ready Stance

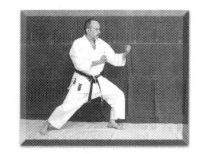

2) Front Foot 1/4 Step Forward Jab
   to Front Stance

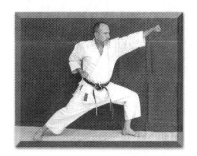

3) Full Step Forward Lunge Punch
   to Front Stance

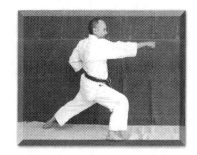

4) Rear Leg Forward 1/2 Step Transition

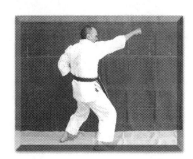

5) Front Leg Forward to Ready Stance

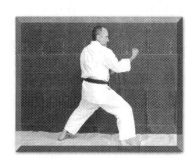

> Kizami Zuki, Oi Zuki

1) Ready Stance

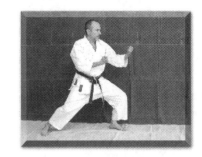

2) Rear Foot 1/2 Step Forward Jab

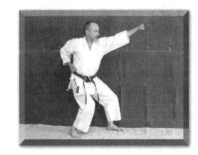

3) Front Foot 1/2 Step Forward
   Reverse Punch to Front Stance

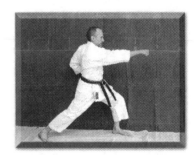

4) Rear Leg Forward 1/2 Step Transition

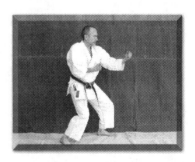

5) Front Leg Forward to Ready Stance

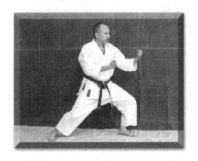

> Kizami Zuki, Gyaku Zuki

Tsuku Kihon 19

1) Ready Stance

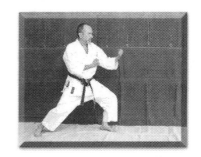

2) Front Foot 1/4 Step Forward
   Reverse Punch to Front Stance

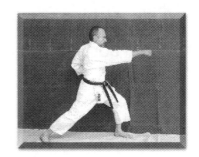

3) Full Step Forward Back Fist Strike
   to Front Stance

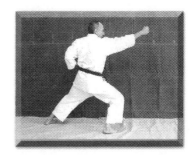

4) Rear Leg Forward 1/2 Step Transition

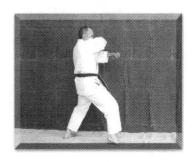

5) Front Leg Forward to Ready Stance

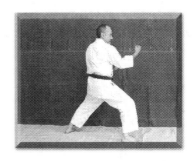

> Gyaku Zuki, Oi Uraken Uchi

Tsuku Kihon 21

1) Ready Stance

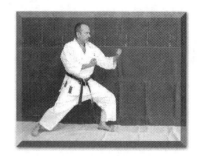

2) Front Foot 1/4 Step Forward
   Reverse Punch to Front Stance

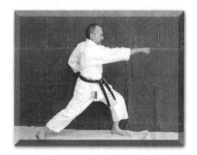

3) Full Step Forward Lunge Punch
   to Front Stance

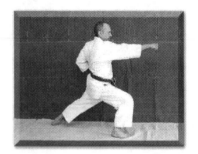

4) Rear Leg Forward 1/2 Step Transition

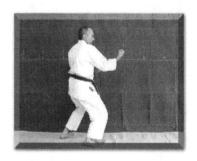

5) Front Leg Forward to Ready Stance

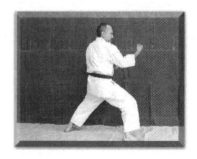

> Gyaku Zuki, Oi Zuki

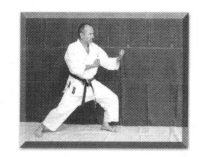

1) Ready Stance

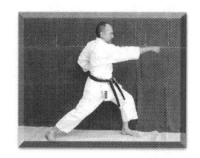

2) Front Foot 1/4 Step Forward
   Reverse Punch to Front Stance

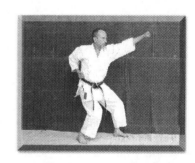

3) Rear Foot 1/2 Step Forward Jab

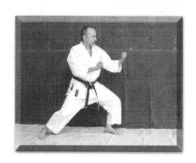

4) Front Foot Step Forward
   to Ready Stance

> Gyaku Zuki, Kizami Zuki

1) Ready Stance

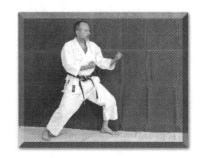

2) Front Foot 1/4 Step Forward
   Reverse Punch to Front Stance

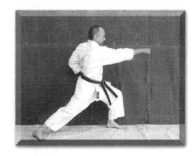

3) Full Step Forward Reverse Punch
   to Front Stance

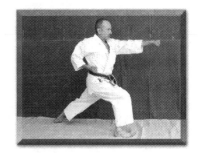

4) Rear Foot 1/2 Step Forward Transition

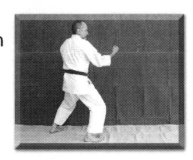

5) Ready Stance

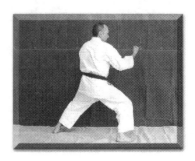

> Gyaku Zuki, Gyaku Zuki

1) Ready Stance

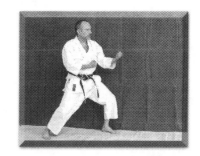

2) Full Step Forward Lunge Punch
   to Front Stance

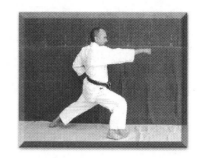

3) Rear Foot 1/2 Step Forward Transition

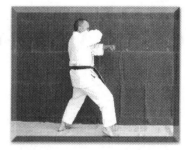

4) Front Foot 1/2 Step Forward
   Back Fist Strike to Front Stance

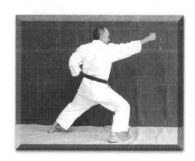

5) Ready Stance

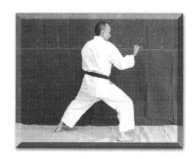

> Oi Zuki, Oi Uraken Uchi

1) Ready Stance

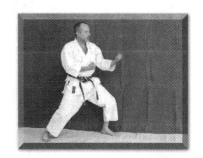

2) Full Step Forward Lunge Punch
   to Front Stance

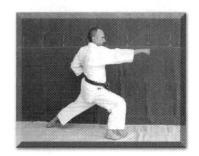

3) Rear Foot 1/2 Step Forward Transition

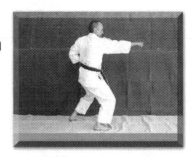

4) Front Foot 1/2 Forward
   Reverse Punch to Front Stance

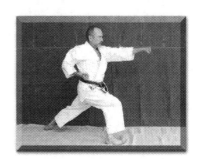

5) Rear Foot Forward to Ready Stance

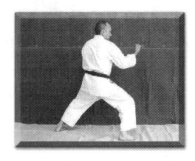

> Oi Zuki, Gyaku Zuki

Tsuku Kihon 26

1) Ready Stance

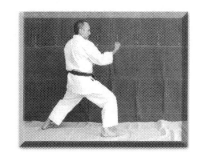

2) Full Step Forward Lunge Punch
   to Front Stance

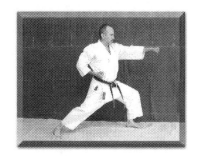

3) Rear Foot 1/2 Step Forward Transition

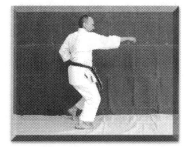

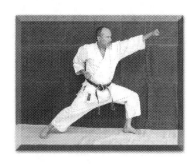

4) Front Foot 1/4 Step Forward Jab
   to Front Stance

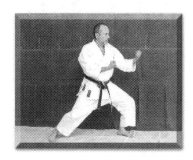

5) Ready Stance

> Oi Zuki, Kizami Zuki

1) Ready Stance

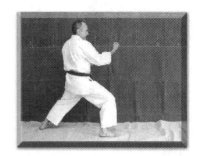

2) Full Step Forward Lunge Punch
   to Front Stance

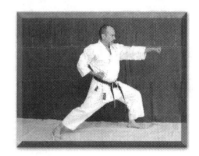

3) Rear Foot 1/2 Step Forward Transition

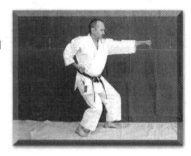

4) Front Foot Snap Kick

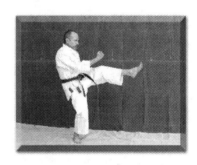

5) Ready Stance

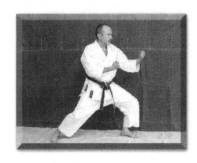

> Oi Zuki, Kizami Mae Geri

Tsuku Kihon 28

1) Ready Stance

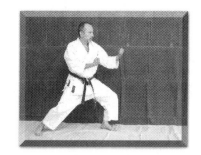

2) Rear Foot Full Step Forward
   Reverse Punch to Front Stance

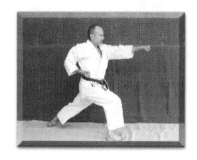

3) Rear Foot 1/2 Step Forward Jab

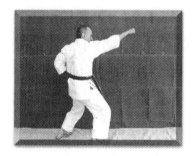

4) Front Foot Step Forward
   to Ready Stance

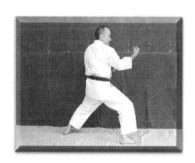

> Kizami Gyaku Zuki, Kizami Zuki

1) Ready Stance

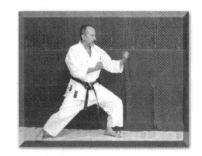

2) Rear Foot Full Step Forward Front
   Hand Reverse Punch to Front Stance

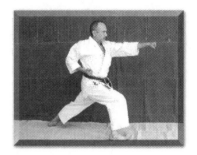

3) Rear Foot 1/2 Step Forward Transition

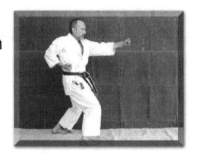

4) Front Foot Forward Lunge Punch
   to Front Stance

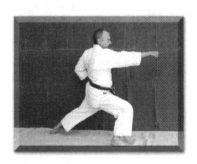

5) Rear Foot 1/4 Step Forward
   to Ready Stance

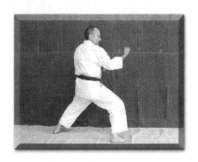

> Kizami Gyaku Zuki, Oi Zuki

1) Ready Stance

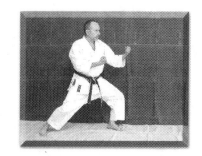

3) Rear Leg Chamber

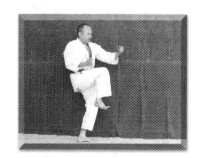

3) Rear Leg Front Snap Kick

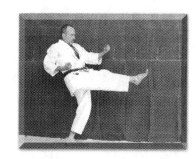

4) Lunge Punch Upon Leg Return
   to Chamber

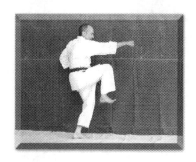

5) Front Leg Forward to Ready Stance

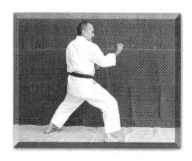

> Gyaku Mae Geri, Oi Zuki

1) Ready Stance

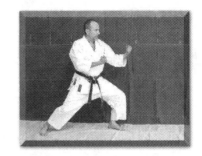

2) Rear Leg Round House Kick

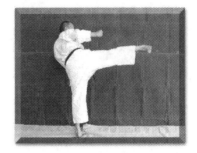

3) Kicking Leg Down to Reverse Punch

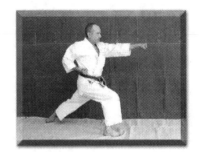

4) Rear Foot 1/2 Step Forward Transition

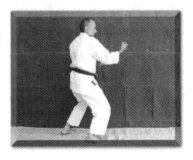

5) Front Leg Forward to Ready Stance

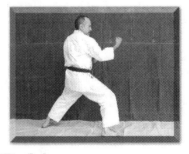

> Gyaku Mawashi Geri, Gyaku Zuki

1) Ready Stance

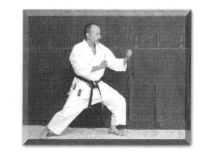

2) Front Leg Chamber

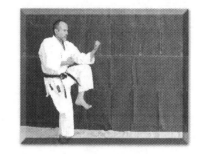

3) Front Leg Snap Kick

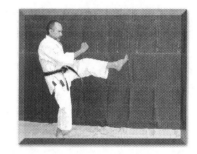

4) Jab As Kicking Leg Retrieves

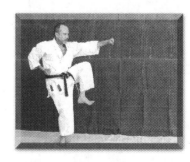

5) Ready Stance

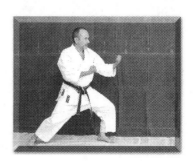

> Kizami Mae Geri, Kizami Zuki

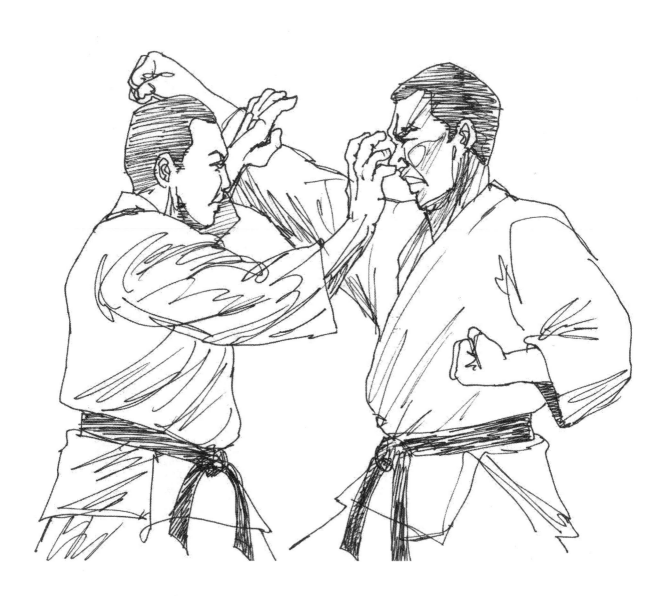

Chapter Six
Triple-Technique Sequence

Starting with triple combinations, rhythm begins to take a much greater role in how techniques are effectively executed. For example, the beat of sequence execution can be: 1 and 2 and 3, or 1-2 and 3, or 1 and 2-3, or 1-2-3. Rhythm depends on variables such as distance to target, reaction from the opponent, and changes in angles to the target. Please note that not all drills listed below are pictured.

o   kamae, front foot ¼ step forward jab, rear foot ½ step forward, front foot ½ step forward reverse punch, rear foot full step forward reverse punch, rear foot ½ step forward, front foot ¼ step forward, kamae **(kizami zuki, gyaku zuki, gyaku zuki)**

o   kamae, front foot ¼ step forward jab, lunge punch to full front stance, rear foot ½ step forward, front foot ¼ step forward reverse punch, rear foot forward ½ step, front foot ¼ step forward, kamae **(kizami zuki, oi zuki, gyaku zuki)**

o   kamae, rear foot ½ step forward jab, front foot ½ step forward reverse punch, rear foot full step forward reverse punch, rear foot ½ step forward, front foot ¼ step forward, kamae **(kizami zuki, gyaku zuki, gyaku zuki)**

o   kamae, front foot ¼ step forward reverse punch, same hand lunge punch to full front stance, rear foot ½ step forward, front foot ¼ step forward reverse punch, rear foot ½ step forward, front foot ¼ step forward, kamae **(gyaku zuki, oi zuki, gyaku zuki)**

o   kamae, front foot ¼ step forward reverse punch, rear foot ½ step forward jab, front foot ½ step forward reverse punch, rear foot ½ step forward, front foot ¼ step forward, kamae **(gyaku zuki, kizami zuki, gyaku zuki)***

o   kamae, lunge punch to full front stance, rear foot ½ step forward, front foot ¼ step forward same hand jab, rear foot ½ step forward, front foot ¼ step forward reverse punch, rear foot ½ step forward, front foot ¼ step forward, kamae **(oi zuki, kizami zuki, gyaku zuki)**

o   kamae, lunge punch to full front stance, rear foot ½ step forward, front foot ½ step forward reverse punch, rear foot full step forward reverse punch, rear foot ½ step forward, front foot ¼ step forward, kamae **(oi zuki, gyaku zuki, gyaku zuki)**

o   kamae, lunge punch to full front stance, rear foot ½ step forward, front foot ½ step forward reverse punch, rear leg front snap kick to full front stance, rear foot ½ step forward, front foot ¼ step forward, kamae **(oi zuki, gyaku zuki, gyaku mae geri)**

o   kamae, rear foot full step forward reverse punch with front hand, rear foot ½ step forward jab, front foot ¼ step forward reverse punch, rear foot forward ½ step, front foot ¼ step forward, kamae **(kizami gyaku zuki, kizami zuki, gyaku zuki)**

o   kamae, rear foot full step forward reverse punch with front hand, same hand lunge punch to full front stance, rear foot ½ step forward, front foot ¼ step forward reverse punch, rear foot ½ step forward, front foot ¼ step forward, kamae **(kizami gyaku zuki, oi zuki, gyaku zuki)**

o   kamae, rear foot full step forward reverse punch with front hand, rear leg round house kick, reverse punch with same hand to full stance, rear foot forward ½ step, front foot ¼ step forward, kamae **(kizami gyaku zuki, gyaku mawashi geri, gyaku zuki)**

o   kamae, rear leg front snap kick, lunge punch to full front stance, rear foot ½ step forward, front foot ¼ step forward reverse punch, rear foot ½ step forward, front foot ¼ step forward, kamae **(gyaku mae geri, oi zuki, gyaku zuki)***

- kamae, front leg snap kick, same side jab, reverse punch to full front stance, front foot back, kamae **(kizami mae geri, kizami zuki, gyaku zuki)**
- kamae, front leg snap kick, kamae, rear leg round house kick, reverse punch to full front stance, rear foot ½ step forward, front foot ¼ step forward, kamae **(kizami mae geri, gyaku mawashi geri, gyaku zuki)**

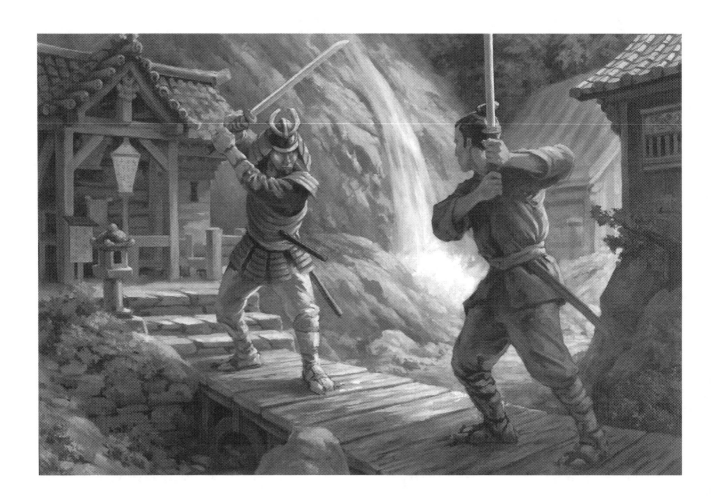

Tsuku Kihon 20

1) Ready Stance

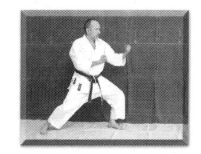

2) Front Foot 1/4 Step Forward Reverse Punch to Front Stance

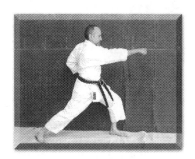

3) Rear Leg Front Snap Kick

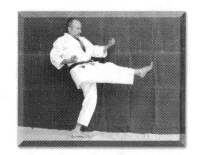

4) Lunge Punch Upon Leg Return to Chamber

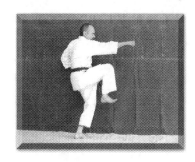

5) Front Leg Forward to Ready Stance

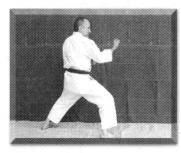

> Gyaku Zuki, Gyaku Mae Geri, Oi Zuki

1) Ready Stance

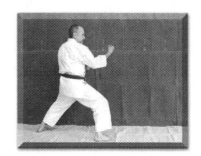

3) Rear Leg Side Thrust Kick

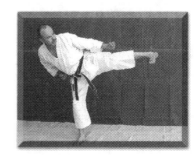

3) Kicking Leg Down to Back Fist Strike

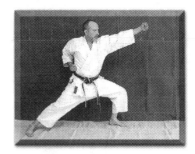

4) Rear Foot 1/2 Step Forward Transition

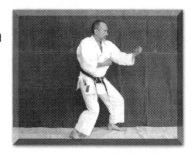

5) Front Leg Forward to Ready Stance

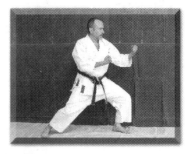

> Gyaku Yoko Geri, Oi Uraken Uchi

1) Ready Stance

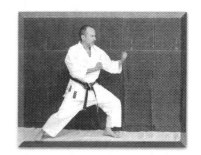

2) Rear Foot 1/2 Step Forward Jab

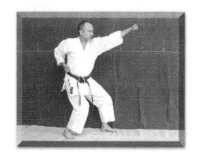

3) Front Foot 1/2 Step Forward Reverse Punch to Front Stance

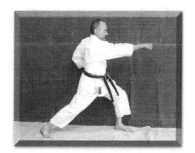

4) Rear Leg Full Step Forward Reverse Punch to Front Stance

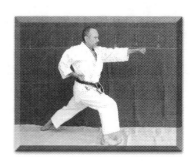

5) Rear Foot Step Forward to Ready Stance

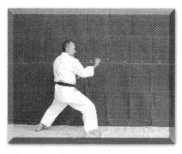

> Kizami Zuki, Gyaku Zuki, Gyaku Zuki

1) Ready Stance

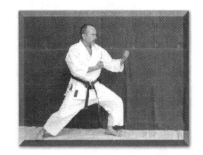

2) Front Foot 1/4 Step Forward
   Reverse Punch to Front Stance

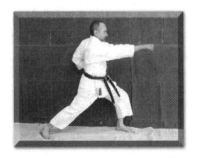

3) Rear Foot 1/2 Step Forward Jab

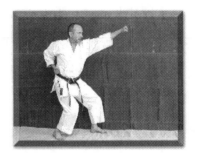

4) Front Foot 1/2 Step Forward
   Reverse Punch to Front Stance

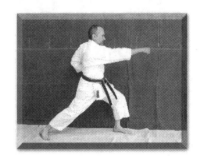

5) Rear Foot Forward to Ready Stance

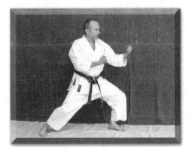

> Gyaku Zuki, Kizami Zuki, Gyaku Zuki

1) Ready Stance

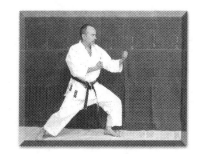

2) Front Leg Snap Kick

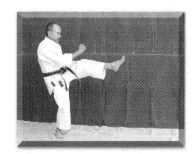

3) Jab As Kicking Leg Retrieves

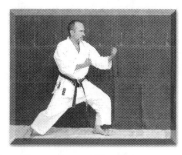

4) Kicking Leg Step Forward
   Reverse Punch to Front Stance

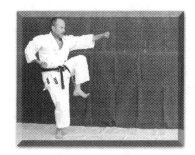

5) Rear Foot Forward to Ready Stance

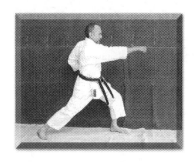

> Kizami Mae Geri, Kizami Zuki, Gyaku Zuki

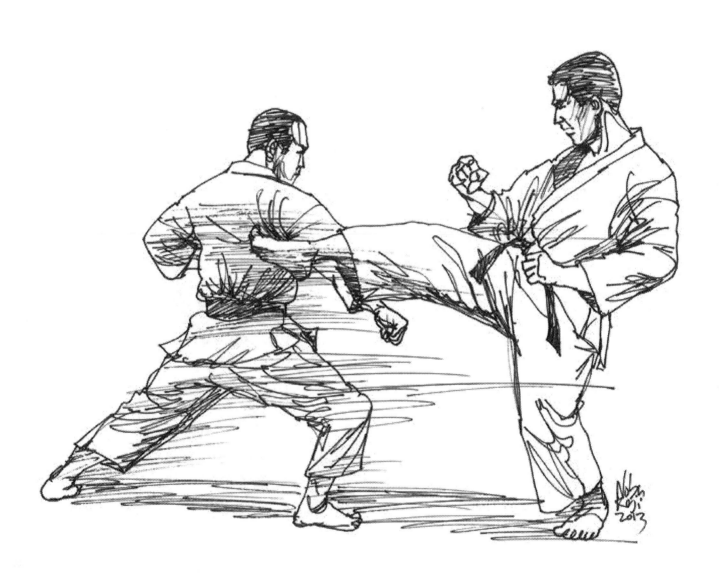

Chapter Seven
Quadruple-Technique Sequence

Please note that not all drills listed below are pictured.

o kamae, front foot ¼ step forward jab, rear foot ½ step forward, front foot ½ step forward reverse punch, rear foot ½ step forward, front foot ¼ step forward, lunge punch to full front stance, rear foot ½ step forward, front foot ½ step forward reverse punch, rear foot ½ step forward, front foot ¼ step forward, kamae **(kizami zuki, gyaku zuki, oi zuki, gyaku zuki)**

o kamae, front foot ¼ step forward jab, rear leg front snap kick, lunge punch to full front stance, rear foot ½ step forward, front foot ¼ step forward, kamae **(kizami zuki, gyaku mae geri, oi zuki, gyaku zuki)**

o kamae, rear foot ½ step forward jab, front foot ½ step forward reverse punch, lunge punch to full front stance, rear foot ½ step forward, front foot ¼ step forward reverse punch, rear foot ½ step forward, front foot ¼ step forward, kamae **(kizami zuki, gyaku zuki, oi zuki, gyaku zuki)**

o kamae, front foot ¼ step forward reverse punch, same hand lunge punch to full front stance, rear foot ½ step forward, same hand jab to full front stance, , rear foot ½ step forward jab, front foot ½ step forward reverse punch rear foot ½ step forward, front foot ¼ step forward, kamae **(gyaku zuki, oi zuki, kizami zuki, gyaku zuki)**

o kamae, front foot ¼ step forward reverse punch, rear leg front snap kick, lunge punch to full front stance, rear foot ½ step forward, front foot ¼ step forward reverse punch, rear foot ½ step forward, front foot ¼ step forward, kamae **(gyaku zuki, gyaku mae geri, oi zuki, gyaku zuki)**

o kamae, front foot ¼ step forward reverse punch, rear foot full step forward reverse punch, rear foot full step forward lunge punch, rear foot ½ step forward, front foot ¼ step forward reverse punch, rear foot ½ step forward, front foot ¼ step forward, kamae **(gyaku zuki, gyaku zuki, oi zuki, gyaku zuki)**

o kamae, lunge punch to full front stance, rear foot ½ step forward, front leg snap kick, same hand lunge jab to full front stance, rear foot ½ step forward, front foot ¼ step forward reverse punch, rear foot ½ step forward, front foot ¼ step forward, kamae **(oi zuki, kizami mae geri, kizami zuki, gyaku zuki)**

o kamae, rear foot full step forward reverse punch with front hand, rear leg front snap kick, lung punch with same hand to full stance, rear foot ½ step forward, front foot ¼ step forward reverse punch, rear foot forward ½ step, front foot ¼ step forward, kamae **(kizami gyaku zuki, gyaku mae geri, oi zuki, gyaku zuki)**

o kamae, front leg snap kick, kamae, rear leg front snap kick, lunge punch to full front stance, rear foot ½ step forward, front foot ¼ step forward reverse punch, rear foot ½ step forward, front foot ¼ step forward, kamae **(kizami mae geri, gyaku mae geri, oi zuki, gyaku zuki)**

1) Ready Stance

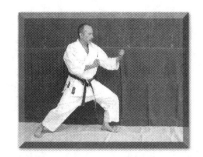

2) Rear Foot 1/2 Step Forward Jab

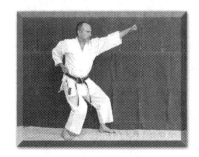

3) Front Foot 1/2 Step Forward
   Reverse Punch to Front Stance

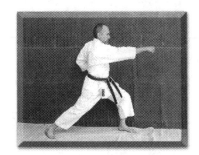

4) Rear Foot Full Step Forward
   Lunge Punch

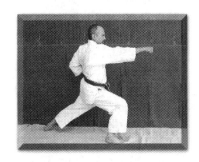

5) Rear Leg 1/2 Step Forward Transition

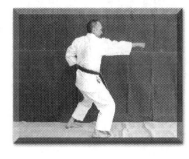

6) Front Leg 1/4 Step Forward
   to Reverse Punch

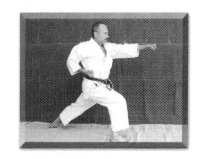

7) Rear Leg 1/2 Step Forward Transition

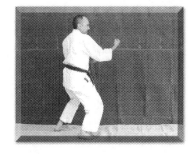

8) Front Leg Forward to Ready Stance

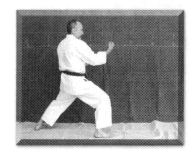

> Kizami Zuki, Gyaku Zuki, Oi Zuki, Gyaku Zuki

1) Ready Stance

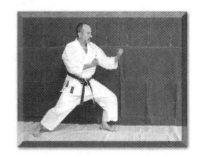

2) Front Foot 1/4 Step Forward
   Reverse Punch to Front Stance

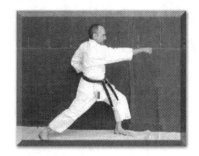

3) Full Step Forward Lunge Punch
   to Front Stance

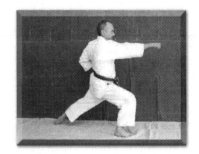

4) Rear Leg Forward 1/2 Step Transition

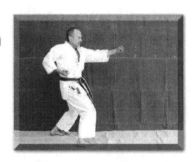

5) Front Leg Forward Verticle Jab
   to Front Stance

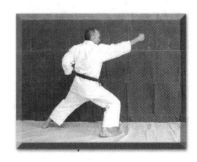

6) Rear Leg Forward 1/2 Step Transition

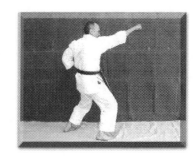

7) Front Foot 1/2 Step Reverse Punch
to Front Stance

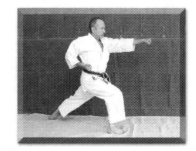

8) Rear Leg Forward 1/2 Step Transition

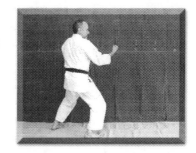

9) Front Leg Step Forward
to Front Stance

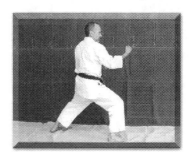

> Gyaku Zuki, Oi Zuki, Kizami Zuki, Gyaku Zuki

1) Ready Stance

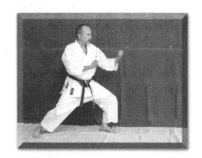

2) Front Foot 1/4 Step Forward
   Reverse Punch to Front Stance

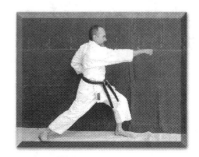

3) Rear Leg Front Snap Kick

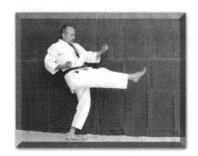

4) Lunge Punch Upon Kicking
   Leg Retrieval

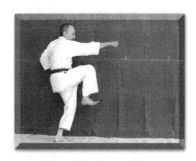

5) Kicking Leg Forward to Front Stance

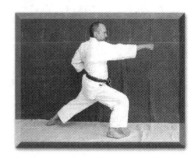

6) Rear Foot Forward 1/2 Step Transition

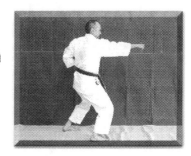

7) Front Foot 1/2 Forward
   Reverse Punch to Front Stance

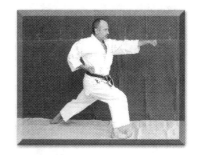

8) Rear Foot 1/2 Step Forward Transition

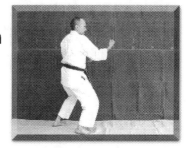

9) Front Foot Step Forward
   to Ready Stance

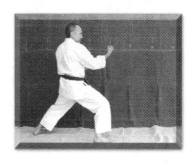

> Gyaku Zuki, Gyaku Mae Geri, Oi Zuki, Gyaku Zuki

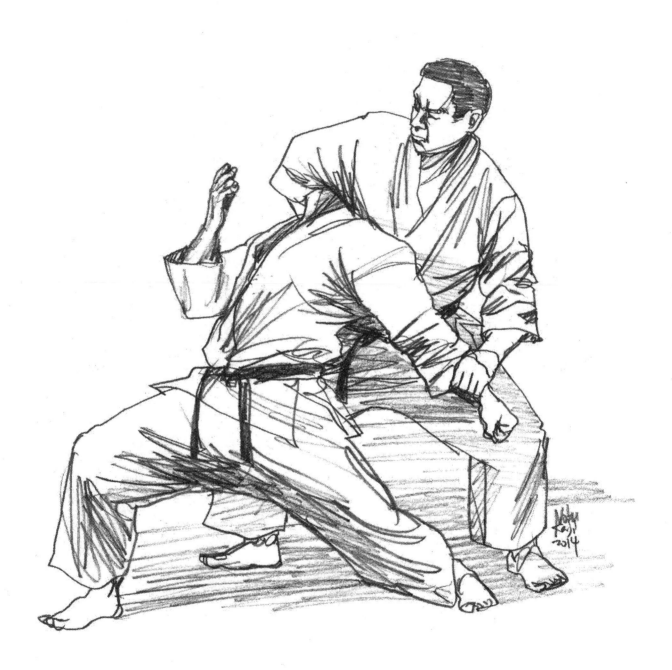

Chapter Eight
Quintuple-Technique Sequence

Please note that not all drills listed below are pictured.

o kamae, front foot ¼ step forward jab, lunge punch to full front stance, rear foot ½ step forward, front foot ¼ step forward reverse punch, lunge punch to full front stance, rear foot ½ step forward, front foot ¼ step forward reverse punch, rear foot ½ step forward, front foot ¼ step forward, kamae **(kizami zuki, oi zuki, gyaku zuki, oi zuki, gyaku zuki)***

o kamae, rear foot ½ step forward jab, front foot ½ step forward reverse punch, rear leg front snap kick, lunge punch to full front stance, rear foot ½ step forward, front foot ¼ step forward reverse punch, rear foot ½ step forward, front foot ¼ step forward, kamae **(kizami zuki, gyaku zuki, gyaku mae geri, oi zuki, gyaku zuki)**

o kamae, rear foot ½ step forward jab, front foot ½ step forward reverse punch, lunge punch to full front stance, rear foot ½ step forward, same hand jab to full front stance, rear foot ½ step forward, front foot ¼ step forward reverse punch, rear foot ½ step forward, front foot ¼ step forward, kamae **(kizami zuki, gyaku zuki, oi zuki, kizami zuki, gyaku zuki)**

o kamae, front foot ¼ step forward reverse punch, rear leg front snap kick, same hand lunge punch to full front stance, rear foot ½ step forward, same hand jab to full front stance, rear foot ½ step forward, front foot ¼ step forward reverse punch, rear foot ½ step forward, front foot ¼ step forward, kamae **(gyaku zuki, gyaku mae geri, oi zuki, kizami zuki, gyaku zuki)**

o kamae, front foot ¼ step forward reverse punch, rear foot full step forward reverse punch, rear leg front snap kick, lunge punch to full front stance, rear foot ½ step forward, front foot ¼ step forward reverse punch, rear foot ½ step forward, front foot ¼ step forward, kamae **(gyaku zuki, gyaku zuki, gyaku mae geri, oi zuki, gyaku zuki)**

o kamae, lunge punch to full front stance, rear foot ½ step forward, front foot ½ step forward reverse punch, rear leg front snap kick, lunge punch to full front stance, rear foot ½ step forward, front foot ¼ step forward reverse punch, rear foot ½ step forward, front foot ¼ step forward, kamae **(oi zuki, gyaku zuki, gyaku mae geri, oi zuki, gyaku zuki)**

o kamae, rear leg front snap kick, lunge punch to full front stance, rear foot ½ step forward, front leg snap kick, same hand jab to full front stance, rear foot ½ step forward, front foot ¼ step forward reverse punch, rear foot ½ step forward, front foot ¼ step forward, kamae **(gyaku mae geri, oi zuki, kizami mae geri, kizami zuki, gyaku zuki)**

Tsuku Kihon 63

1) Ready Stance

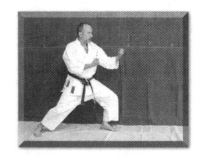

2) Front Foot 1/4 Step Forward
   Reverse Punch to Front Stance

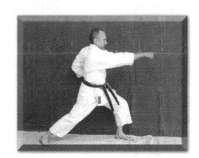

3) Full Step Forward Reverse Punch
   to Front Stance

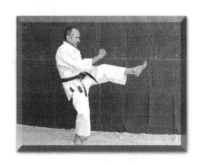

4) Rear Leg Front Snap Kick

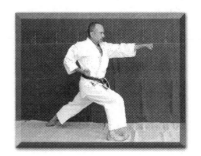

5) Lunge Punch At the Same Time
   Kicking Leg Retrieves

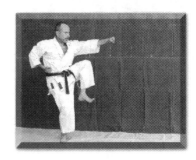

6) Kicking Foot Forward to Front Stance

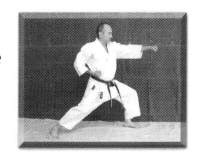

7) Rear Foot 1/2 Step Forward Transition

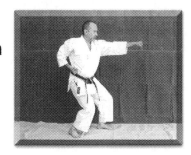

8) Front 1/2 Step Foot Forward
   Reverse Punch to Front Stance

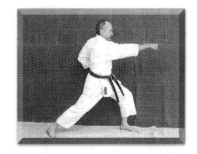

9) Rear Foot Step Forward
   to Ready Stance

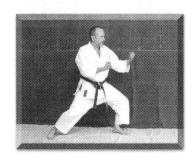

> Gyaku Zuki, Gyaku Zuki, Gyaku Mae Geri, Oi Zuki, Gyaku Zuki

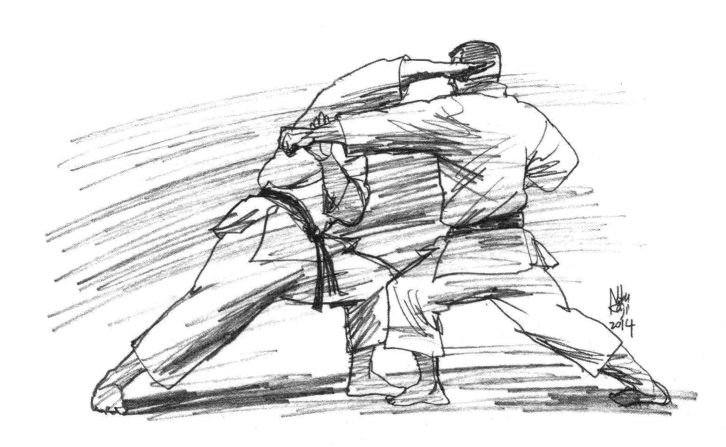

Chapter Nine
Sextuple-Technique Sequence

Combinations of six techniques, in my view, are the maximum practical number that can be strung together, otherwise things simply become repetitive. Please note that not all drills listed below are pictured.

- kamae, front leg snap kick, same side jab, reverse punch to full front stance, rear leg front snap kick, lunge punch to full front stance, rear foot ½ step forward, front foot ¼ step forward reverse punch, rear foot ½ step forward, front foot ¼ step forward, kamae (**kizami mae geri, kizami zuki, gyaku zuki, gyaku mae geri, oi zuki, gyaku zuki**)
- kamae, front foot ¼ step forward reverse punch, rear leg front snap kick, lunge punch to full front stance, rear foot ½ step forward, front leg snap kick, same hand jab to full front stance, rear foot ½ step forward, front foot ¼ step forward reverse punch, rear foot ½ step forward, front foot ¼ step forward, kamae (**gyaku zuki, gyaku mae geri, oi zuki, kizami mae geri, kizami zuki, gyaku zuki**)

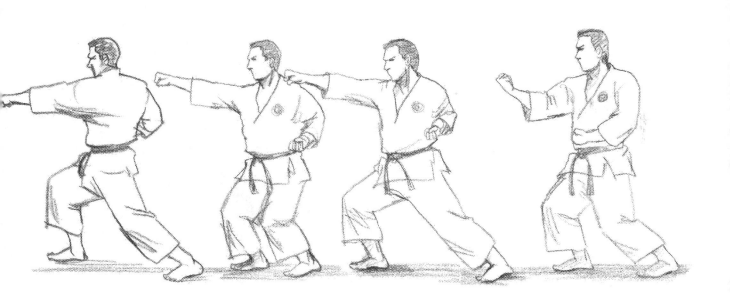

Tsuku Kihon 67

1) Ready Stance

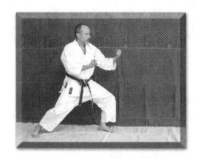

2) Front Foot 1/4 Step Forward
   Reverse Punch to Front Stance

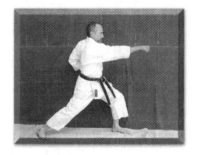

3) Rear Leg Front Snap Kick

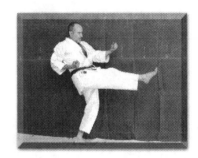

4) Lunge Punch to Full Front Stance

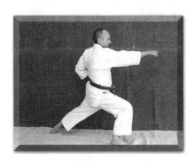

5) Rear Leg Half Step Forward

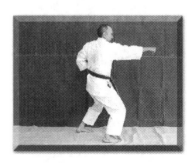

Tsuku Kihon 67

6) Front Leg Snap Kick

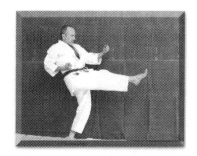

7) Jab At the Same Time Kicking
   Leg Retrieves

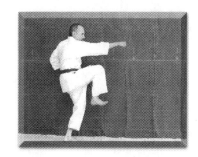

8) Rear Leg 1/2 Step Foot Forward
   Reverse Punch to Front Stance

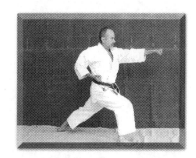

9) Rear Foot Step Forward
   to Ready Stance

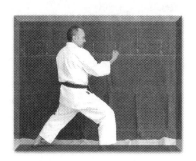

> Gyaku Zuki, Gyaku Mae Geri, Oi Zuki,
  Kizami Mae Geri, Kizami Zuki, Gyaku Zuki

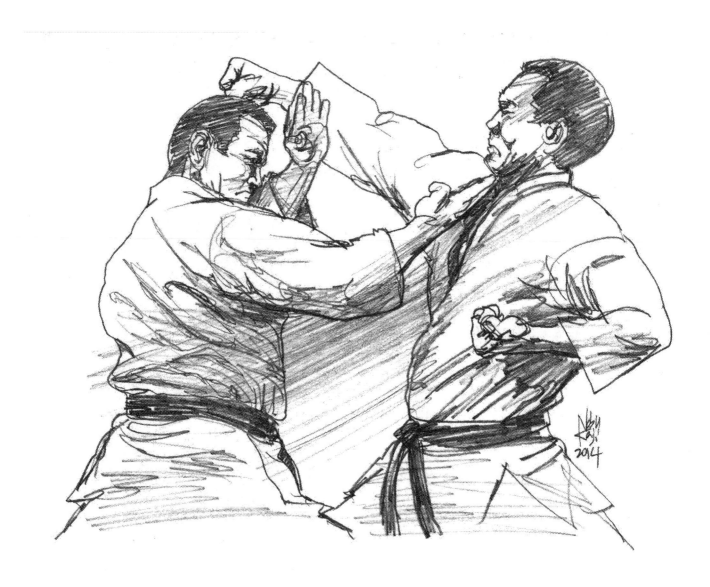

Chapter Ten
Heavy Bag Training

Once Tsuku Kihon techniques are understood fairly well, it's time to use them against the heavy bag. Doing so will teach proper distance to the target so that maximum penetrating power can be achieved. The following sets should first be performed from stationary kamae to achieve consistent stances at the point of impact.

Start out by doing Tsuku Kihon exactly as executed during normal drills. Every technique must be fully extended and complete. Stances must also be settled into and complete. Make distance adjustments so maximum power and penetration into the bag is achieved.

Combinations will need to be executed rapidly because the bag moves when hit and there is little time to complete subsequent techniques. That is why three-technique combinations are the practical limit for proper execution and penetration into the bag.

After practicing stationary Tsuku Kihon with the heavy bag for a few weeks, the next step is to execute techniques from a free-sparring mobile stance. Treat the heavy bag as a live target and move in using Tsuku Kihon and move back out to kamae. This is a great way to develop zanshin and to practice techniques against a moving target. Techniques will now need to be snappy and drawn back fast, though still complete. In other words, the length of time that a technique is held in the complete and extended position is much shorter than when doing normal drills. Please note that not all drills listed below are pictured.

a. kamae, front foot ¼ step forward jab, front foot back, kamae **(kizami zuki)***
b. kamae, front foot ¼ step forward jab, rear foot ½ step forward, step back, kamae **(kizami zuki)**
c. kamae, rear foot ½ step forward jab, rear foot ½ step back, kamae **(kizami zuki)***
d. kamae, rear foot ½ step forward jab, front foot ½ step forward, step back, kamae **(kizami zuki)***
e. kamae, front foot ¼ step forward reverse punch, front foot back, kamae **(gyaku zuki)***
f. kamae, front foot ¼ step forward reverse punch, rear foot ½ step forward, step back, kamae **(gyaku zuki)**
g. kamae, front foot ¼ step forward reverse punch, rear foot step 45 degrees to side, step back, kamae **(oi gyaku zuki)**
h. kamae, front foot ¼ step forward back fist to full front stance, front foot back, kamae **(kizami uraken uchi)**
i. kamae, lunge punch to full front stance, step back, kamae **(oi zuki)**
j. kamae, lunge punch to full front stance, rear foot ½ step forward, step back, kamae **(oi zuki)**
k. kamae, lunge back fist to full front stance, rear foot ½ step forward, step back, kamae **(oi uraken uchi)**
l. kamae, rear foot full step forward reverse punch with front hand, rear foot forward ½ step, step back, kamae **(kizami gyaku zuki)**
m. kamae, front foot ¼ step forward jab, rear foot ½ step forward, front foot ½ step forward reverse punch, step back, kamae **(kizami zuki, gyaku zuki)***

n. kamae, front foot ¼ step forward jab, reverse punch, bring front foot back, kamae **(kizami zuki, gyaku zuki)**

o. kamae, rear foot ½ step forward jab, front foot ½ step forward reverse punch, step back, kamae **(kizami zuki, gyaku zuki)**

p. kamae, front foot ¼ step forward reverse punch, rear foot ½ step forward jab, step back, kamae **(gyaku zuki, kizami zuki)**

q. kamae, front foot ¼ step forward reverse punch, rear foot 45 degree side step jab, step back, kamae **(gyaku zuki, kizami zuki)**

r. kamae, front foot ¼ step forward reverse punch, rear foot full step forward reverse punch, step back, kamae **(gyaku zuki, gyaku zuki)**

s. kamae, lunge punch to full front stance, rear foot ½ step forward, front foot ¼ step forward reverse punch, step back, kamae **(oi zuki, gyaku zuki)**

t. kamae, lunge punch to full front stance, front foot ¼ step forward same hand jab, step back, kamae **(oi zuki, kizami zuki)**

u. kamae, rear foot full step forward reverse punch with front hand, rear foot ½ step forward jab, step back, kamae **(kizami gyaku zuki, kizami zuki)**

v. kamae, rear foot full step forward reverse punch with front hand, rear foot 45 degree side step jab, step back, kamae **(kizami gyaku zuki, kizami zuki)**

w. kamae, rear leg front snap kick, lunge punch to full front stance, step back, kamae **(gyaku mae geri, oi zuki)**

x. kamae, rear leg round house kick, reverse punch to full front stance, step back, kamae **(gyaku mawashi geri, gyaku zuki)**

y. kamae, front foot ¼ step forward reverse punch, rear leg round house kick, step back, kamae **(gyaku zuki, gyaku mawashi geri)***

z. kamae, rear leg side thrust kick, lunge back fist to full front stance, step back, kamae **(gyaku yoko geri, oi uraken uchi)**

aa. kamae, rear leg spinning back kick, reverse punch to full front stance, step back, kamae **(uchiro geri, gyaku zuki)**

bb. kamae, rear leg front snap kick, lunge back fist to full front stance, step back, kamae **(gyaku mae geri, oi uraken uchi)***

cc. kamae, front leg snap kick, same side jab to full front stance, front foot back, kamae **(kizami mae geri, kizami zuki)**

dd. kamae, front foot ¼ step forward reverse punch, rear foot ½ step forward jab, front foot ½ step forward reverse punch, step back, kamae **(gyaku zuki, kizami zuki, gyaku zuki)***

ee. kamae, rear foot full step forward reverse punch with front hand, rear foot ½ step forward jab, front foot ¼ step forward reverse punch, step back, kamae **(kizami gyaku zuki, kizami zuki, gyaku zuki)**

ff. kamae, front leg snap kick, same side jab, reverse punch to full front stance, front foot back, kamae **(kizami mae geri, kizami zuki, gyaku zuki)**

gg. kamae, rear foot full step forward lunge punch, rear foot ½ step forward, front foot ¼ step forward reverse punch, rear foot 45 degrees side step jab, kamae **(oi zuki, gyaku zuki, kizami zuki)**

hh. kamae, front foot ¼ step forward reverse punch, rear foot 45 degree side step jab, front foot step forward gyaku zuki, step back, kamae **(gyaku zuki, kizami zuki, gyaku zuki)**

Heavy Bag Drill B

1) Kamae

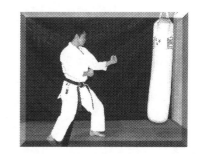

2) Front Foot Forward Jab
   to Front Stance

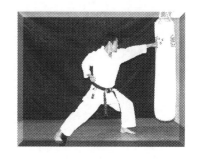

3) Rear Foot Half Step Forward

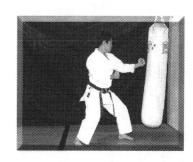

4) Step Back to Kamae

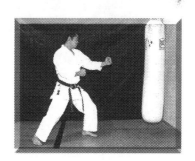

> Kizami Zuki

Heavy Bag Drill C

1) Kamae

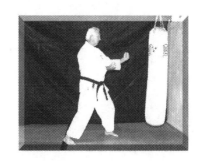

2) Rear Foot Half Step Forward Jab

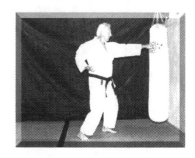

3) Rear Foot Back to Kamae

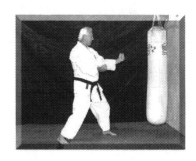

> Kizami Zuki

Heavy Bag Drill F

1) Kamae

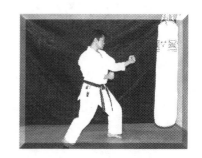

2) Front Foot Forward Reverse Punch
   to Front Stance

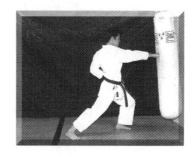

3) Rear Foot Half Step Forward

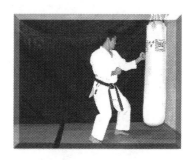

4) Step Back to Kamae

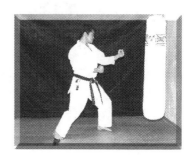

> Gyaku Zuki

Heavy Bag Drill G

1) Kamae

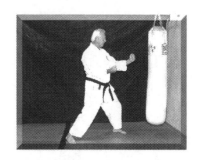

2) Front Foot Forward Reverse Punch
   to Front Stance

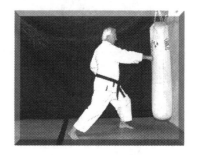

3) Rear Foot Shift 45 Degrees to Kamae

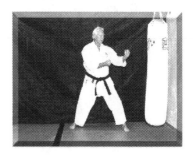

4) Step Back to Kamae

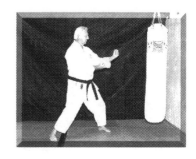

> Gyaku Zuki

Heavy Bag Drill H

1) Kamae

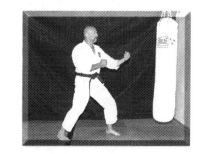

2) Front Foot Stepping Forward
   Striking Chamber Arm

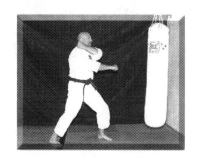

3) Front Foot Continue Forward
   Back Fist to Front Stance

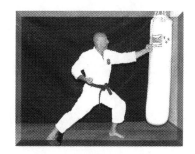

4) Re-Chamber Striking Arm

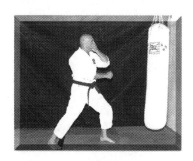

5) Step Back to Kamae

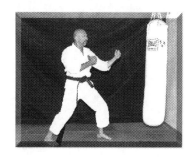

> Kizami Uraken Ushi

Heavy Bag Drill I

1) Kamae

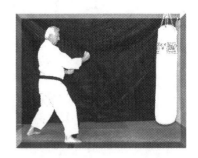

2) Rear Foot Full Step Forward
   Lunge Punch to Front Stance

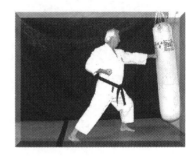

3) Front Foot Back to Kamae

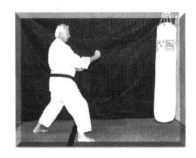

> Oi Zuki

Heavy Bag Drill J

1) Kamae

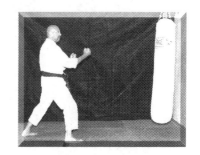

2) Rear Foot Full Step Forward Lunge
   Punch to Front Stance

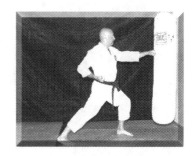

3) Rear Foot Half Step Forward

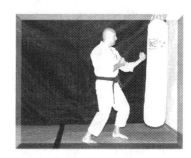

4) Step Back to Kamae

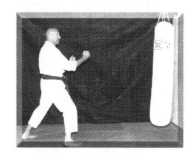

> Oi Zuki

Heavy Bag Drill L

1) Kamae

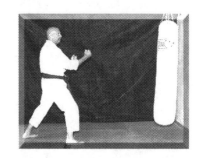

2) Rear Foot Full Step Forward Front
   Hand Reverse Punch to Front Stance

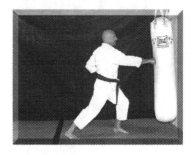

3) Rear Foot Half Step Forward

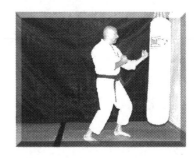

4) Step Back to Kamae

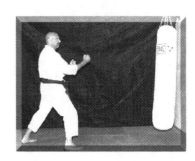

> Kizami Gyaku Zuki

Heavy Bag Drill M

1) Kamae

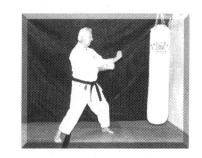

2) Front Foot Step Forward Jab
   to Front Stance

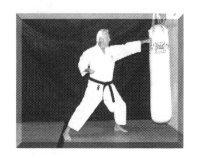

3) Rear Foot Half Step Forward

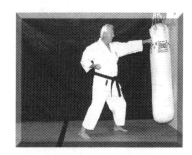

4) Front Foot Step Forward Reverse
   Punch to Front Stance

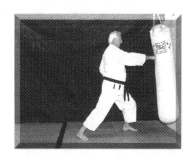

5) Step Back to Kamae

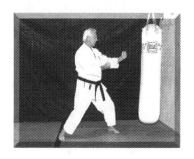

> Kizami Zuki, Gyaku Zuki

Heavy Bag Drill N

1) Kamae

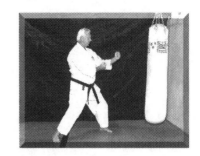

2) Front Foot Forward Jab
   to Front Stance

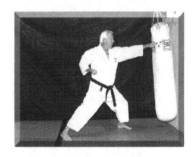

3) Reverse Punch

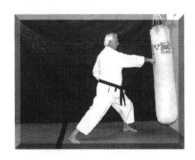

4) Step Back to Kamae

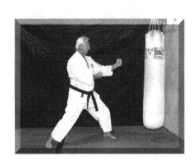

> ## Kizami Zuki, Gyaku Zuki

Heavy Bag Drill O

1) Kamae

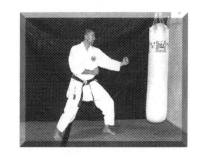

2) Rear Foot Half Step Forward Jab

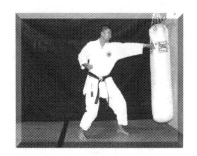

3) Front Foot Step Forward Reverse
   Punch to Front Stance

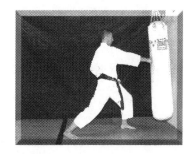

4) Step Back to Kamae

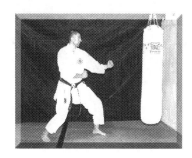

> Kizami Zuki, Gyaku Zuki

Heavy Bag Drill Q

1) Kamae

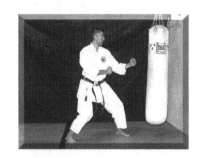

2) Front Foot Step Forward Reverse Punch to Front Stance

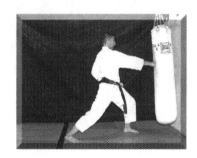

3) Rear Foot Side Step 45 Degrees Jab to Front Stance

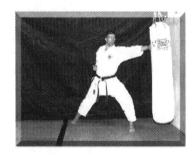

4) Step Back to Kamae

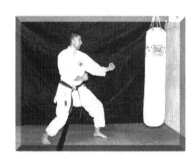

> Gyaku Zuki, Kizami Zuki

Heavy Bag Drill R

1) Kamae

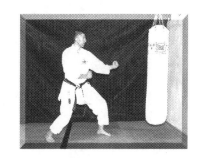

2) Front Foot Step Forward Reverse Punch to Front Stance

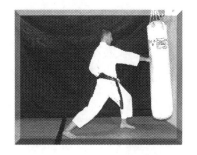

3) Front Foot Shift Back, Rear Foot Full Step Forward Reverse Punch to Front Stance

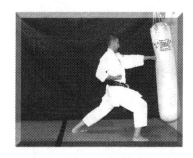

4) Step Back to Kamae

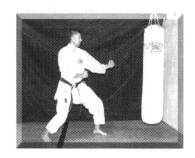

> Gyaku Zuki, Gyaku Zuki

Heavy Bag Drill S

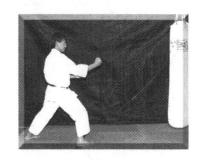

1) Kamae

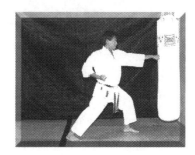

2) Rear Foot Full Step Forward Lunge Punch to Front Stance

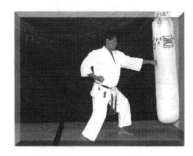

3) Rear Foot Half Step Forward

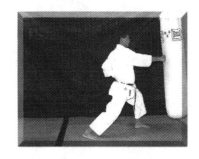

4) Front Foot Step Forward Reverse Punch to Front Stance

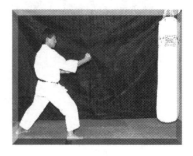

5) Step Back to Kamae

> Oi Zuki, Gyaku Zuki

Heavy Bag Drill T

1) Kamae

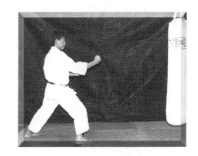

2) Rear Foot Full Step Forward Lunge
   Punch to Front Stance

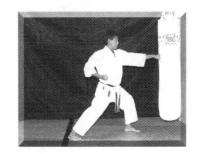

3) Rear Foot Half Step Forward,
   Chamber Arm That Just Punched

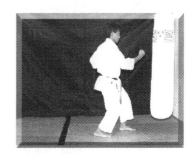

4) Front Foot Step Forward Jab

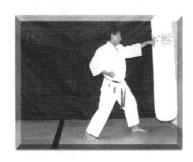

5) Step Back to Kamae

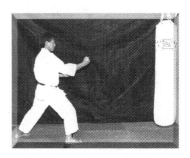

> Oi Zuki, Kizami Zuki

Heavy Bag Drill V

1) Kamae

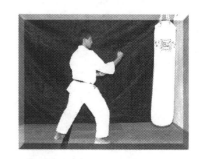

2) Rear Foot Full Step Forward Front Hand Reverse Punch to Front Stance

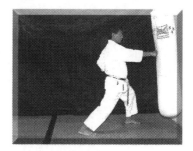

3) Rear Foot Shift 45 Degrees Jab to Front Stance

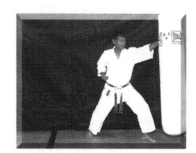

4) Step Back to Kamae

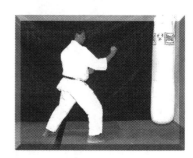

> Kizami Gyaku Zuki, Kizami Zuki

Heavy Bag Drill W

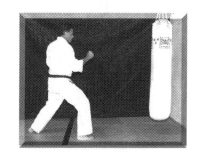

1) Kamae

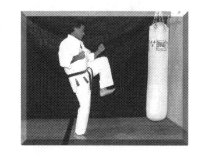

2) Rear Foot Front Snap Kick Chamber

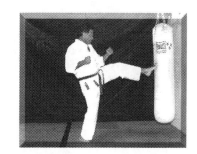

3) Front Snap Kick

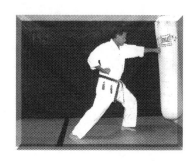

4) Lunge Punch As Kicking Foot
   Retrieves to Front Stance

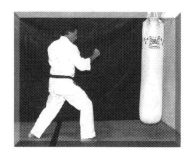

5) Step Back to Kamae

> Gyaku Mae Geri, Oi Zuki

Heavy Bag Drill X

1) Kamae

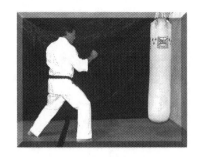

2) Rear Foot Front Round House
   Kick Chamber

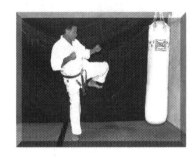

3) Round House Kick

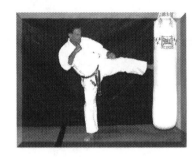

4) Reverse Punch As Kicking Foot
   Retrieves to Front Stance

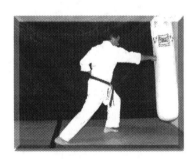

5) Step Back to Kamae

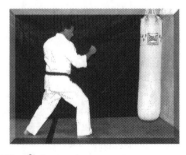

> Gyaku Mawashi Geri, Gyaku Zuki

Heavy Bag Drill Y

1) Kamae

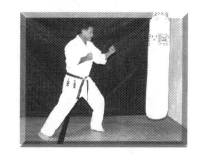

2) Front Foot Forward Reverse Punch to Front Stance

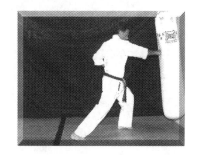

3) Rear Foot Front Round House Kick Chamber

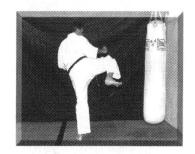

4) Round House Kick

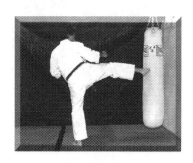

5) Step Back to Kamae

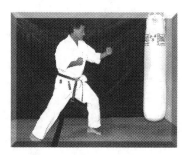

> Gyaku Zuki, Gyaku Mawashi Geri

Heavy Bag Drill Z

1) Kamae

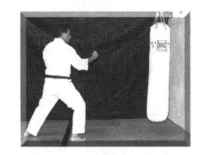

2) Rear Foot Side Thrust Kick Chamber

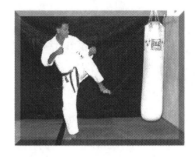

3) Side Thrust Kick

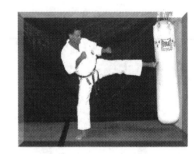

4) Back Fist Strike as Kicking Leg
   Retrieves to Front Stance

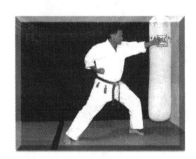

5) Step Back to Kamae

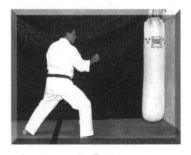

> Gyaku Yoko Geri Keikome, Uraken Ushi

Heavy Bag Drill AA

1) Kamae

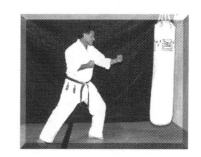

2) Spinning Back Kick Chamber

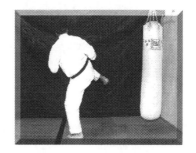

3) Spinning Back Kick

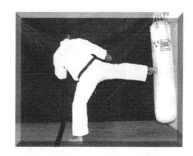

4) Reverse Punch as Kicking Leg Retrieves to Front Stance

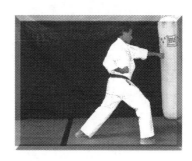

5) Step Back to Kamae

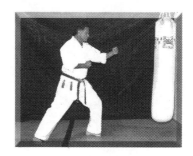

> Ushiro Geri, Gyaku Zuki

Heavy Bag Drill CC

1) Kamae

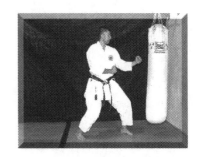

2) Front Foot Snap Kick

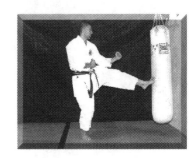

3) Jab At the Same Time Kicking
   Leg Retrieves

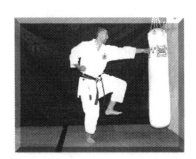

4) Front Foot Step Forward to Kamae

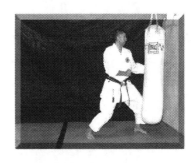

5) Step Back to Kamae

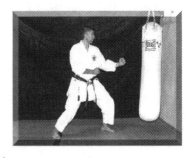

> Kizami Mae Geri, Kizami Zuki

Heavy Bag Drill DD

1) Kamae

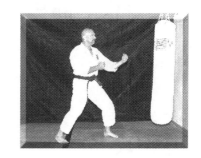

2) Front Foot Step Forward Reverse Punch to Front Stance

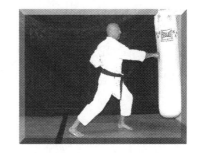

3) Rear Foot Quarter Step Forward Jab

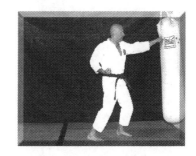

4) Front Foot Step Forward Reverse Punch to Front Stance

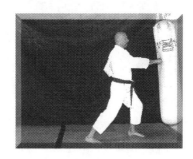

5) Step Back to Kamae

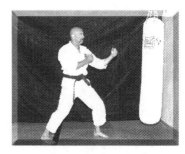

> Gyaku Zuki, Kizami Zuki, Gyaku Zuki

Heavy Bag Drill EE

1) Kamae

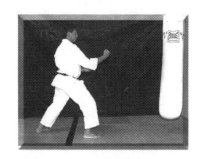

2) Rear Foot Full Step Forward Front Hand Reverse Punch to Front Stance

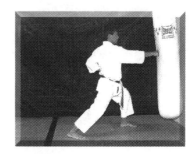

3) Rear Foot Half Step Forward Jab

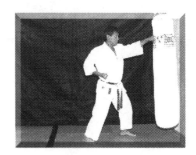

4) Front Foot Step Forward Reverse Punch to Front Stance

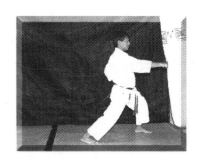

5) Step Back to Kamae

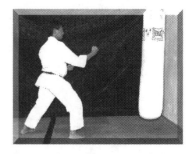

> Kizami Gyaku Zuki, Kizami Zuki, Gyaku Zuki

Heavy Bag Drill FF

1) Kamae

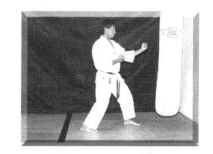

2) Front Foot Snap Kick

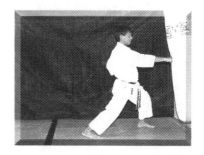

3) Jab At the Same Time Foot Retrieves

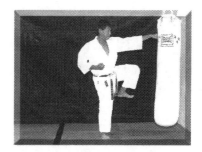

4) Front Foot Step Forward Reverse Punch to Front Stance

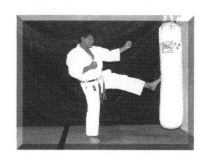

5) Step Back to Kamae

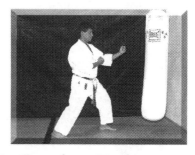

> Kizami Mae Geri, Kizami Zuki, Gyaku Zuki

Heavy Bag Drill GG

1) Kamae

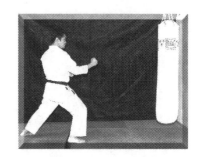

2) Rear Foot Full Step Forward Lunge
   Punch to Front Stance

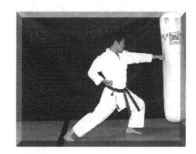

3) Front Foot Thrust Forward
   Reverse Punch

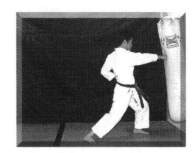

4) Rear Foot 45 Degrees Side Step Jab

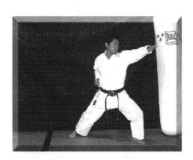

5) Step Back to Kamae

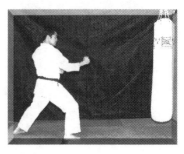

> Oi Zuki, Gyaku Zuki, Kizami Zuki

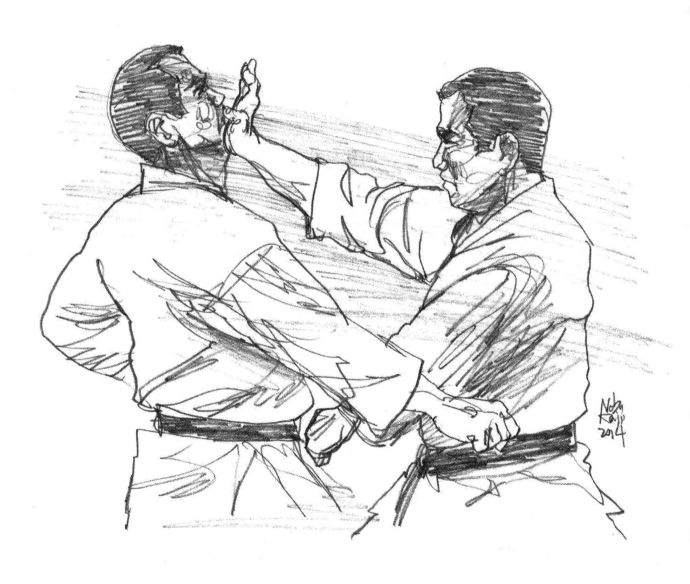

Chapter Eleven
Makiwara Training

Practicing Tsuku Kihon with the makiwara is similar to the techniques used on the heavy bag. The main difference is that combinations are limited to two techniques each. Because the makiwara is stiff and yields only slightly, care should be taken to prevent injuries to the hands and arm joints.

Makiwara training is a great way to develop compression of muscles at the point of impact. Proper distance is crucial so corrections need to happen quickly, as must fist, wrist and forearm alignment. Also, because the makiwara is a small target, its use will improve accuracy as well. Please note that not all drills listed below are pictured.

a. kamae, front foot ¼ step forward jab, front foot back, kamae **(kizami zuki)***
b. kamae, front foot ¼ step forward jab, rear foot ½ step forward, step back, kamae **(kizami zuki)**
c. kamae, rear foot ½ step forward jab, rear foot ½ step back, kamae **(kizami zuki)***
d. kamae, rear foot ½ step forward jab, front foot ½ step forward, step back, kamae **(kizami zuki)***
e. kamae, shift weight forward reverse punch, shift weight back, kamae **(gyaku zuki)**
f. kamae, front foot ¼ step forward reverse punch, front foot back, kamae **(gyaku zuki)***
g. kamae, front foot ¼ step forward reverse punch, rear foot ½ step forward, step back, kamae **(gyaku zuki)**
h. kamae, front foot ¼ step forward reverse punch, rear foot side step 45 degrees, step back, kamae **(oi gyaku zuki)**
i. kamae, lunge punch to full front stance, rear foot ½ step forward, step back, kamae **(oi zuki)**
j. kamae, rear foot full step forward reverse punch with front hand, rear foot forward ½ step, step back, kamae **(kizami gyaku zuki)**
k. kamae, front foot ¼ step forward jab, then reverse punch, bring front foot back, kamae **(kizami zuki, gyaku zuki)**
l. kamae, rear foot ½ step forward jab, front foot ½ step forward reverse punch, step back, kamae **(kizami zuki, gyaku zuki)**
m. kamae, front foot ¼ step forward reverse punch, rear foot ½ step forward jab, step back, kamae **(gyaku zuki, kizami zuki)**
n. kamae, rear foot full step forward reverse punch with front hand, rear foot ½ step forward jab, step back, kamae **(kizami gyaku zuki, kizami zuki)**
o. kamae, lunge punch to full front stance, then reverse punch, step back, kamae **(oi zuki, gyaku zuki)**
p. kamae, lunge punch to full front stance, rear foot ½ step forward reverse punch, step back, kamae **(oi zuki, gyaku zuki)**
q. kamae, side thrust kick to full front stance, reverse punch, step back, kamae **(yoko geri keikome, gyaku zuki)**
r. kamae, rear leg half step reverse punch, step back, kamae **(gyaku zuki)**

Makiwara Drill A

1) Kamae

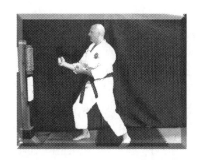

2) Front Foot Step Forward Jab
   to Front Stance

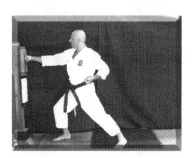

3) Front Leg Back to Kamae

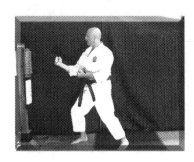

> Kizami Zuki

Makiwara Drill E

1) Kamae With Weight Shifted Back

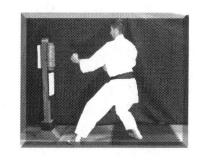

2) Shift Weight Forward to Front Stance Reverse Punch

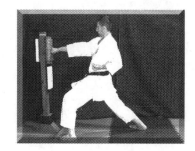

3) Shift Weight Back to Kamae

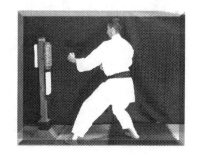

> Gyaku Zuki

Makiwara Drill F

1) Kamae

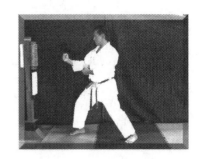

2) Front Foot Step Forward Reverse
   Punch to Front Stance

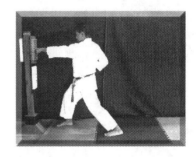

3) Front Foot Back to Kamae

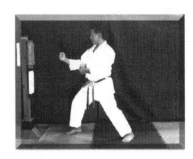

> Gyaku Zuki

Makiwara Drill M

1) Kamae

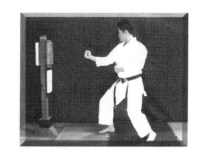

2) Front Foot Forward Reverse Punch to Front Stance

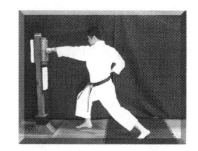

3) Rear Foot Half Step Forward Jab

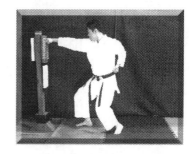

4) Step Back to Kamae

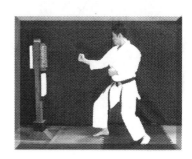

> Gyaku Zuki, Kizami Zuki

Makiwara Drill N

1) Kamae

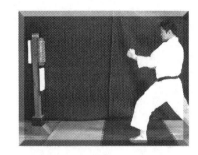

2) Rear Foot Full Step Forward Reverse
   Punch with Front Hand to Front Stance

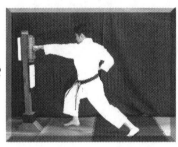

3) Rear Foot Half Step Forward Jab

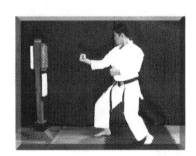

4) Step Back to Kamae

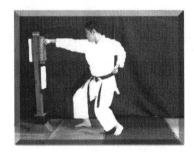

> Kizami Gyaku Zuki, Kizami Zuki

Makiwara Drill Q

1) Kamae

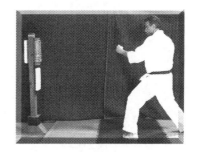

2) Rear Leg Side Thrust Kick Chamber

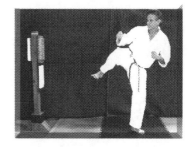

3) Side Thurst Kick

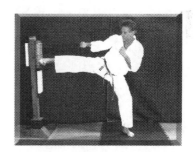

4) Reverse Punch As Kicking Leg
   Re-Chambers and Drops

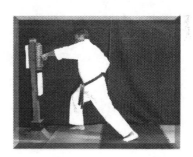

5) Kamae

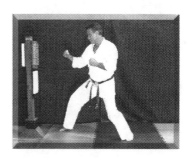

> Gyaku Yoko Geri Keikome, Gyaku Zuki

Makiwara Drill R

1) Kamae

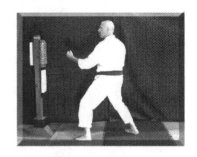

2) Rear Foot Half Step Forward
    Reverse Punch

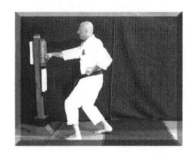

3) Rear Foot Back to Kamae

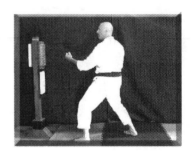

> Gyaku Zuki

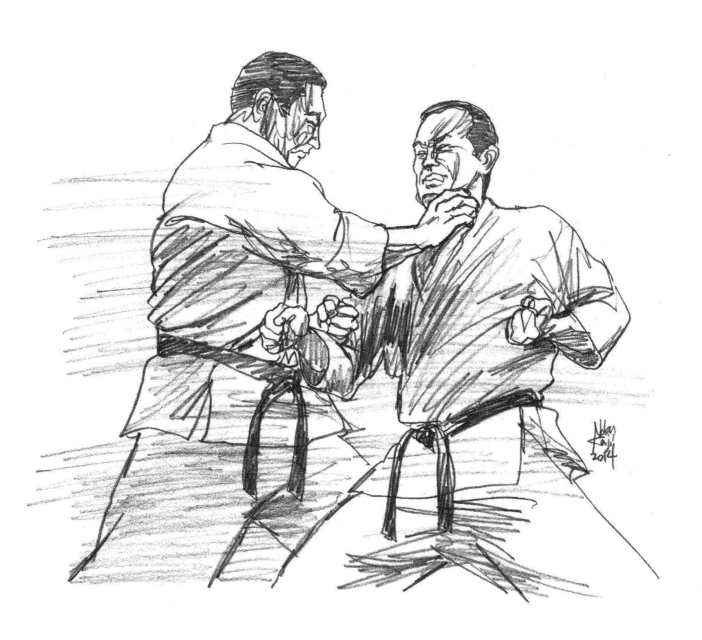

Chapter Twelve
Applications

Tsuku Kihon is particularly effective when executed by children against bullies or people bigger than them. Because kids are usually smaller than the attacker, they must effectively use their body mass and proper technique to maximize impact on the opponent. Therefore, in the following pages, young karateka Sophia and Dominic Mercado demonstrate practical application of select Tsuku Kihon techniques.

Angles using Tsuku Kihon vary depending on how fast an opponent comes in and how close you wish to be to the attacker. In general, most blocks and counter attacks are at a 45-degree angle. If the attacker has a long reach or is very quick and moves very close to you, the counter-attack may end up being at 90 degrees or more to the target. Whichever angle it turns out to be, the important thing is that the direction of the counter-attack be perpendicular to the target so that maximum power is achieved.

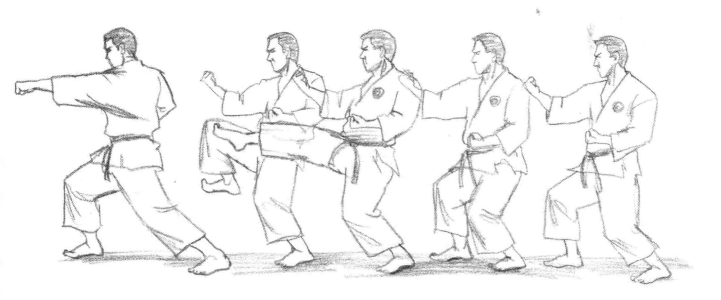

Tsuku Bunaki Set A

1) Natural ready stance.

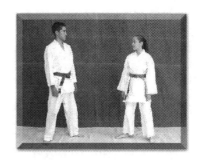

2) Front leg forward jab to front stance at the instant the attacker moves.

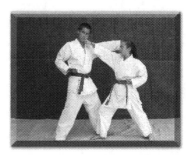

3) Front leg back to ready stance.

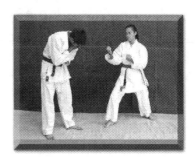

Tsuku Bunkai Set B

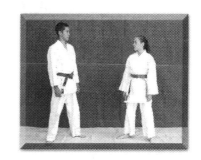

1) Natural ready stance.

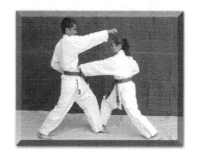

2) Front leg forward reverse punch to front stance at the instant the attacker moves.

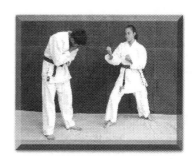

3) Front leg back to ready stance.

Tsuku Bunkai Set C

1) Fighting stance.

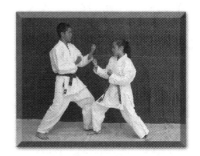

2) Rear foot forward half step jab the instant the attacker moves forward.

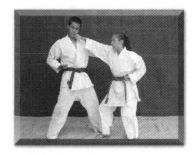

3) Rear foot back to ready stance.

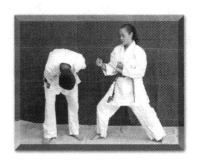

Tsuku Bunkai Set D

1) Natural ready stance.

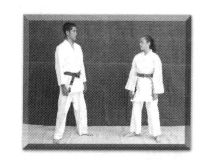

2) Front foot forward back fist strike the instant the attacker moves.

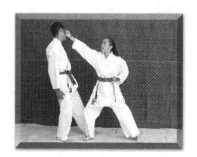

3) Rear foot back to ready stance.

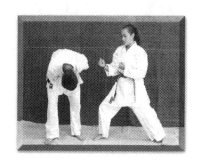

Tsuku Bunkai Set E

1) Natural ready stance.

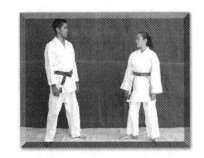

2) Front leg forward jab to front stance the instant the attacker moves, rear leg shifts 45' at same time.

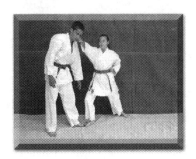

3) Front leg back to ready stance.

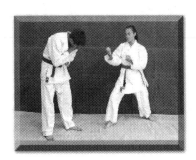

Tsuku Bunkai Set F

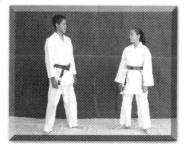

1) Natural ready stance.

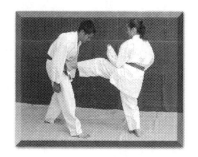

2) Defender kicks with rear leg at the instant opponent attacks, defender will step left.

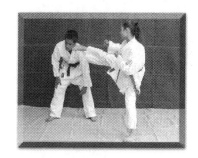

3) As soon as defender steps left she executes a roundhouse kick to the opponent's jaw.

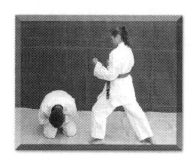

4) Defender steps back into ready position.

Tsuku Bunkai Set G

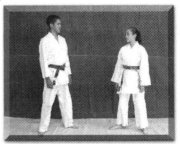

1) Natural ready stance.

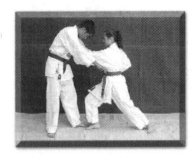

2) Defender reverse punches at the instant opponent attacks.

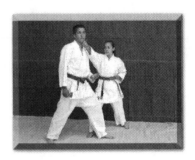

3) Defender steps right with rear leg and at the same time jabs to the opponent's jaw.

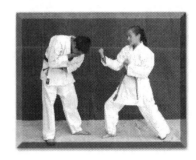

4) Defender steps back into ready position.

Tsuku Bunkai Set H

1) Natural ready stance.

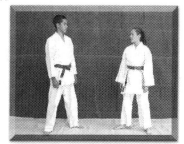

2) Defender reverse punches at the instant opponent attacks.

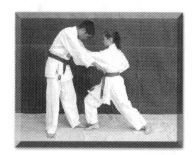

3) Defender steps forward with rear leg and at the same time jabs to the opponent's throat.

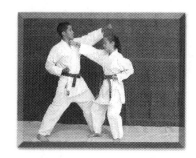

4) Defender steps back into ready position.

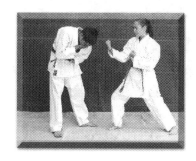

Tsuku Bunkai Set 1

1) Natural ready stance.

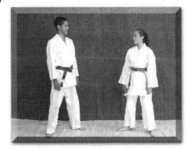

2) Defender blocks at the instant the opponent attacks.

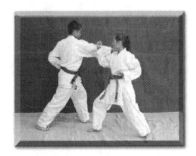

3) Defender reverse punches to the opponent's jaw.

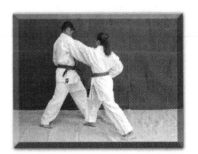

4) Defender steps back into ready position.

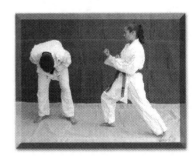

Tsuku Bunkai Set J

1) Natural ready stance.

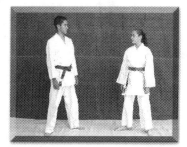

2) Defender step to side at the instant the opponent attacks.

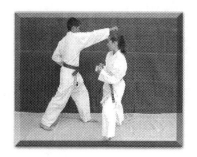

3) Defender side thrust kick to the opponent's knee.

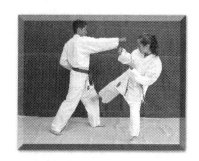

4) Defender steps back into ready position.

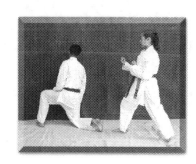

Tsuku Bunkai Set K

1) Natural ready stance.

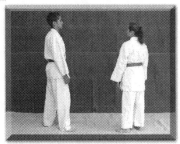

2) Defender kicks groin at the instant the opponent attacks.

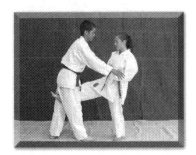

3) Defender executes elbow strike to the opponent's jaw.

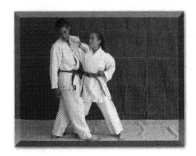

4) Defender steps back into ready position.

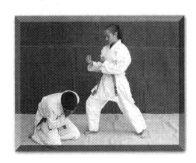

Tsuku Bunkai Set L

1) Natural ready stance.

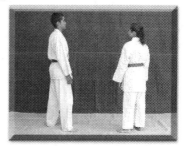

2) Defender steps to side and thrust kicks to knee at the instant opponent attacks.

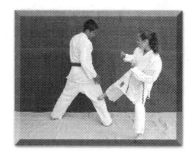

3) Defender reverse punches to the opponent's jaw.

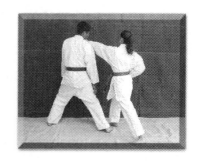

4) Defender steps back into ready position.

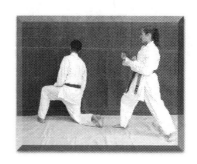

Tsuku Bunkai Set M

1) Natural ready stance.

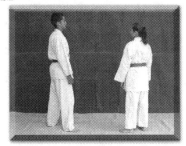

2) Defender kicks with front foot to solar plexus at the instant opponent attacks.

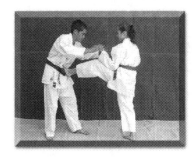

3) Defender reverse spear hand to the opponent's throat.

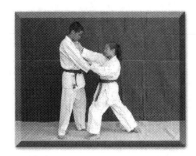

4) Defender steps back into ready position.

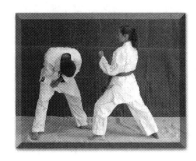

Tsuku Bunkai Set N

1) Natural ready stance.

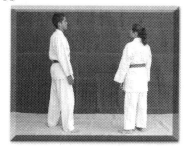

2) Defender thrust kicks with rear foot to the stomach at the instant opponent attacks.

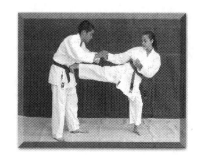

3) Defender reverse punch to the opponent's solar plexus.

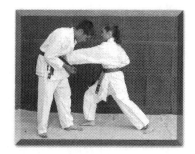

4) Defender steps back into ready position.

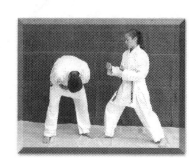

Tsuku Bunkai Set O

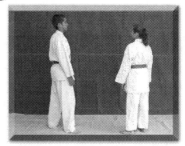

1) Natural ready stance.

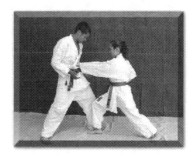

2) Defender reverse punch to stomach at the instant opponent attacks.

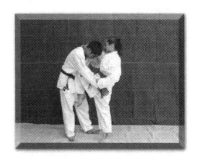

3) Defender knee strike to the opponent's solar plexus.

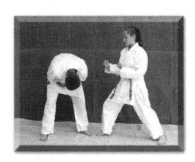

4) Defender steps back into ready position.

Tsuku Bunkai Set P

1) Natural ready stance.

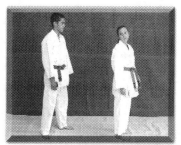

2) Defender side thrust kick to stomach at the instant opponent attacks.

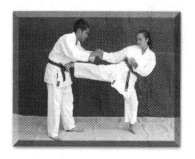

3) Defender back fist strike to the opponent's temple.

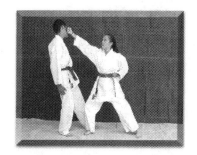

4) Defender steps back into ready position.

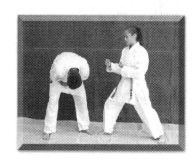

Tsuru Bunkai Set Q

1) Natural ready stance.

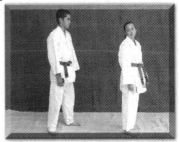

2) Defender turns and grabs arm at the instant the opponent attacks.

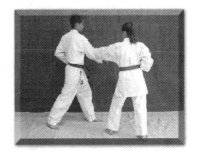

3) Defender thursts arm to opponent's neck.

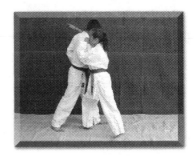

4) Defender slips behind opponent and applies rear naked choke.

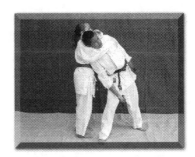

5) Defender releases unconsious opponent and gets to ready stance.

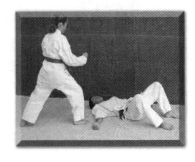

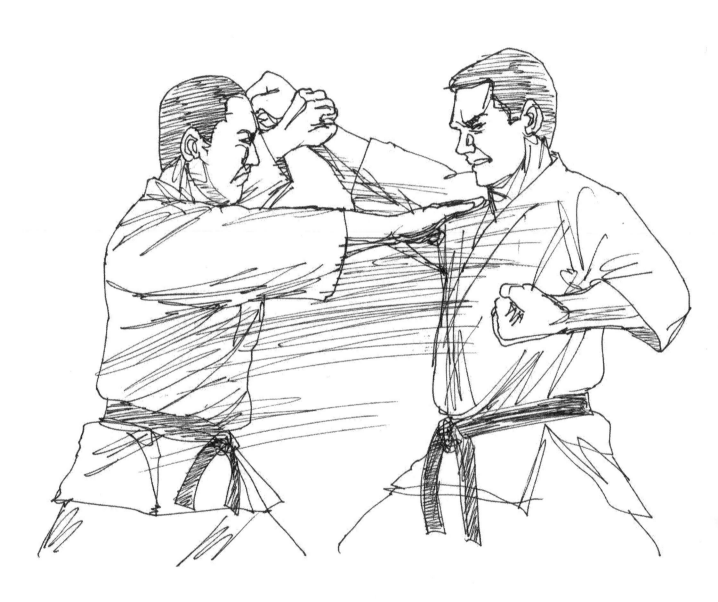

162

Chapter Thirteen
Variations in Training Order

Tsuku Kihon can be taught in several different sequences depending on goals. I have found that varying the order of practice helps keep training interesting and makes one's mind and body more adaptable to changes in real combat and sparring. Practicing one set during one training session is a terrific cardio workout and helps sharpen technique and rhythm.

Sequential

1) kamae, front foot ¼ step forward jab, front foot back, kamae **(kizami zuki)***
2) kamae, front foot ¼ step forward jab, rear foot ½ step forward, front foot ¼ step forward, kamae **(kizami zuki)***
3) kamae, rear foot ½ step forward jab, rear foot ½ step back, kamae **(kizami zuki)***
4) kamae, rear foot ½ step forward jab, front foot ½ step forward, kamae **(kizami zuki)***
5) kamae, front foot ¼ step forward reverse punch, front foot back, kamae **(gyaku zuki)***
6) kamae, front foot ¼ step forward reverse punch, rear foot ½ step forward, front foot ¼ step forward, kamae **(gyaku zuki)***
7) kamae, front foot ¼ step forward reverse punch, rear foot full step forward, kamae **(oi gyaku zuki)***
8) kamae, front foot ¼ step forward back fist to full front stance, front foot back, kamae **(kizami uraken uchi)**
9) kamae, front foot ¼ step forward back fist to full front stance, rear foot ½ step forward, front foot ¼ step forward, kamae **(kizami uraken uchi)**
10) kamae, lunge punch to full front stance, rear foot ½ step forward, front foot ¼ step forward, kamae **(oi zuki)***
11) kamae, lunge back fist to full front stance, rear foot ½ step forward, front foot ¼ step forward, kamae **(oi uraken uchi)***
12) kamae, rear foot full step forward reverse punch with front hand, rear foot forward ½ step, front foot ¼ step forward, kamae **(kizami gyaku zuki)**
13) kamae, front foot ¼ step forward jab, rear foot ½ step forward, front foot ½ step forward reverse punch, rear foot ½ step forward, front foot ¼ step forward, kamae **(kizami zuki, gyaku zuki)***
14) kamae, front foot ¼ step forward jab, reverse punch, bring front foot back, kamae **(kizami zuki, gyaku zuki)**
15) kamae, rear foot ½ step forward jab, rear foot ½ step back reverse punch, kamae **(kizami zuki, gyaku zuki)**
16) kamae, front foot ¼ step forward jab, lunge punch to full front stance, rear foot ½ step forward, front foot ¼ step forward, kamae **(kizami zuki, oi zuki)***
17) kamae, rear foot ½ step forward jab, front foot ½ step forward reverse punch, rear foot ½ step forward, front foot ¼ step forward, kamae **(kizami zuki, gyaku zuki)**
18) kamae, rear foot ½ step forward reverse punch, rear foot ½ step back jab, kamae **(gyaku zuki, kizami zuki)**
19) kamae, front foot ¼ step forward reverse punch, same hand lunge back fist to full front stance, rear foot ½ step forward, front foot ¼ step forward, kamae **(gyaku zuki, oi uraken uchi)***

20) kamae, front foot ¼ step forward reverse punch, rear leg front snap kick, rear foot ½ step forward, front foot ¼ step forward, kamae **(gyaku zuki, gyaku mae geri)*

21) kamae, front foot ¼ step forward reverse punch, same hand lunge punch to full front stance, rear foot ½ step forward, front foot ¼ step forward, kamae **(gyaku zuki, oi zuki)**

22) kamae, front foot ¼ step forward reverse punch, rear foot ½ step forward jab, front foot ¼ step forward, kamae **(gyaku zuki, kizami zuki)**

23) kamae, front foot ¼ step forward reverse punch, rear foot full step forward reverse punch, rear foot ½ step forward, front foot ¼ step forward, kamae **(gyaku zuki, gyaku zuki)*

24) kamae, lunge punch to full front stance, rear foot ½ step forward, front foot ¼ step forward same hand back fist, kamae **(oi zuki, oi uraken uchi)*

25) kamae, lunge punch to full front stance, rear foot ½ step forward, front foot ¼ step forward reverse punch, rear foot ½ step forward, front foot ¼ step forward, kamae **(oi zuki, gyaku zuki)*

26) kamae, lunge punch to full front stance, rear foot ½ step forward, front foot ¼ step forward same hand jab, rear foot ½ step forward, front foot ¼ step forward, kamae **(oi zuki, kizami zuki)*

27) kamae, lunge punch to full front stance, rear foot ½ step forward, front leg front snap kick to full front stance, rear foot ½ step forward, front foot ¼ step forward, kamae **(oi zuki, kizami mae geri)**

28) kamae, rear foot full step forward reverse punch with front hand, rear foot ½ step forward jab, front foot ¼ step forward, kamae **(kizami gyaku zuki, kizami zuki)**

29) kamae, rear foot full step forward reverse punch with front hand, same hand lunge punch to full front stance, rear foot ½ step forward, front foot ¼ step forward, kamae **(kizami gyaku zuki, oi zuki)**

30) kamae, rear leg front snap kick, lunge punch to full front stance, rear foot ½ step forward, front foot ¼ step forward, kamae **(gyaku mae geri, oi zuki)*

31) kamae, rear leg round house kick, reverse punch to full front stance, rear foot ½ step forward, front foot ¼ step forward, kamae **(gyaku mawashi geri, gyaku zuki)*

32) kamae, rear leg side thrust kick, lunge back fist to full front stance, rear foot ½ step forward, front foot ¼ step forward, kamae **(gyaku yoko geri, oi uraken uchi)*

33) kamae, rear leg spinning back kick, reverse punch to full front stance, rear foot ½ step forward, front foot ¼ step forward, kamae **(uchiro geri, gyaku zuki)*

34) kamae, rear leg front snap kick, lunge back fist to full front stance, rear foot ½ step forward, front foot ¼ step forward, kamae **(gyaku mae geri, oi uraken uchi)*

35) kamae, front leg snap kick, same side jab to full front stance, front foot back, kamae **(kizami mae geri, kizami zuki)**

36) kamae, front foot ¼ step forward jab, rear foot ½ step forward, front foot ½ step forward reverse punch, rear foot full step forward reverse punch, rear foot ½ step forward, front foot ¼ step forward, kamae **(kizami zuki, gyaku zuki, gyaku zuki)**

37) kamae, front foot ¼ step forward jab, lunge punch to full front stance, rear foot ½ step forward, front foot ¼ step forward reverse punch, rear foot forward ½ step, front foot ¼ step forward, kamae **(kizami zuki, oi zuki, gyaku zuki)**

38) kamae, rear foot ½ step forward jab, front foot ½ step forward reverse punch, rear foot full step forward reverse punch, rear foot ½ step forward, front foot ¼ step forward, kamae **(kizami zuki, gyaku zuki, gyaku zuki)**

39) kamae, front foot ¼ step forward reverse punch, same hand lunge punch to full front stance, rear foot ½ step forward, front foot ¼ step forward reverse punch, rear foot ½ step forward, front foot ¼ step forward, kamae **(gyaku zuki, oi zuki, gyaku zuki)**

40) kamae, front foot ¼ step forward reverse punch, rear foot ½ step forward jab, front foot ½ step forward reverse punch, rear foot ½ step forward, front foot ¼ step forward, kamae **(gyaku zuki, kizami zuki, gyaku zuki)***

41) kamae, lunge punch to full front stance, rear foot ½ step forward, front foot ¼ step forward same hand jab, rear foot ½ step forward, front foot ¼ step forward reverse punch, rear foot ½ step forward, front foot ¼ step forward, kamae **(oi zuki, kizami zuki, gyaku zuki)**

42) kamae, lunge punch to full front stance, rear foot ½ step forward, front foot ½ step forward reverse punch, rear foot full step forward reverse punch, rear foot ½ step forward, front foot ¼ step forward, kamae **(oi zuki, gyaku zuki, gyaku zuki)**

43) kamae, lunge punch to full front stance, rear foot ½ step forward, front foot ½ step forward reverse punch, rear leg front snap kick to full front stance, rear foot ½ step forward, front foot ¼ step forward, kamae **(oi zuki, gyaku zuki, gyaku mae geri)**

44) kamae, rear foot full step forward reverse punch with front hand, rear foot ½ step forward jab, front foot ¼ step forward reverse punch, rear foot forward ½ step, front foot ¼ step forward, kamae **(kizami gyaku zuki, kizami zuki, gyaku zuki)**

45) kamae, rear foot full step forward reverse punch with front hand, same hand lunge punch to full front stance, rear foot ½ step forward, front foot ¼ step forward reverse punch, rear foot ½ step forward, front foot ¼ step forward, kamae **(kizami gyaku zuki, oi zuki, gyaku zuki)**

46) kamae, rear foot full step forward reverse punch with front hand, rear leg round house kick, reverse punch with same hand to full stance, rear foot forward ½ step, front foot ¼ step forward, kamae **(kizami gyaku zuki, gyaku mawashi geri, gyaku zuki)**

47) kamae, rear leg front snap kick, lunge punch to full front stance, rear foot ½ step forward, front foot ¼ step forward reverse punch, rear foot ½ step forward, front foot ¼ step forward, kamae **(gyaku mae geri, oi zuki, gyaku zuki)***

48) kamae, front leg snap kick, same side jab, reverse punch to full front stance, front foot back, kamae **(kizami mae geri, kizami zuki, gyaku zuki)**

49) kamae, front leg snap kick, kamae, rear leg round house kick, reverse punch to full front stance, rear foot ½ step forward, front foot ¼ step forward, kamae **(kizami mae geri, gyaku mawashi geri, gyaku zuki)**

50) kamae, front foot ¼ step forward jab, rear foot ½ step forward, front foot ½ step forward reverse punch, rear foot ½ step forward, front foot ¼ step forward, lunge punch to full front stance, rear foot ½ step forward, front foot ½ step forward reverse punch, rear foot ½ step forward, front foot ¼ step forward, kamae **(kizami zuki, gyaku zuki, oi zuki, gyaku zuki)**

51) kamae, front foot ¼ step forward jab, rear leg front snap kick, lunge punch to full front stance, rear foot ½ step forward, front foot ¼ step forward, kamae **(kizami zuki, gyaku mae geri, oi zuki, gyaku zuki)**

52) kamae, rear foot ½ step forward jab, front foot ½ step forward reverse punch, lunge punch to full front stance, rear foot ½ step forward, front foot ¼ step forward reverse punch, rear foot ½ step forward, front foot ¼ step forward, kamae **(kizami zuki, gyaku zuki, oi zuki, gyaku zuki)**

53) kamae, front foot ¼ step forward reverse punch, same hand lunge punch to full front stance, rear foot ½ step forward, same hand jab to full front stance, , rear foot ½ step forward jab, front foot ½ step forward reverse punch rear foot ½ step forward, front foot ¼ step forward, kamae **(gyaku zuki, oi zuki, kizami zuki, gyaku zuki)**

54) kamae, front foot ¼ step forward reverse punch, rear leg front snap kick, lunge punch to full front stance, rear foot ½ step forward, front foot ¼ step forward reverse punch, rear foot ½ step forward, front foot ¼ step forward, kamae **(gyaku zuki, gyaku mae geri, oi zuki, gyaku zuki)**

55) kamae, front foot ¼ step forward reverse punch, rear foot full step forward reverse punch, rear foot full step forward lunge punch, rear foot ½ step forward, front foot ¼ step forward reverse

punch, rear foot ½ step forward, front foot ¼ step forward, kamae **(gyaku zuki, gyaku zuki, oi zuki, gyaku zuki)**

56) kamae, lunge punch to full front stance, rear foot ½ step forward, front leg snap kick, same hand lunge jab to full front stance, rear foot ½ step forward, front foot ¼ step forward reverse punch, rear foot ½ step forward, front foot ¼ step forward, kamae **(oi zuki, kizami mae geri, kizami zuki, gyaku zuki)**

57) kamae, rear foot full step forward reverse punch with front hand, rear leg front snap kick, lung punch with same hand to full stance, rear foot ½ step forward, front foot ¼ step forward reverse punch, rear foot forward ½ step, front foot ¼ step forward, kamae **(kizami gyaku zuki, gyaku mae geri, oi zuki, gyaku zuki)**

58) kamae, front leg snap kick, kamae, rear leg front snap kick, lunge punch to full front stance, rear foot ½ step forward, front foot ¼ step forward reverse punch, rear foot ½ step forward, front foot ¼ step forward, kamae **(kizami mae geri, gyaku mae geri, oi zuki, gyaku zuki)**

59) kamae, front foot ¼ step forward jab, lunge punch to full front stance, rear foot ½ step forward, front foot ¼ step forward reverse punch, lunge punch to full front stance, rear foot ½ step forward, front foot ¼ step forward reverse punch, rear foot ½ step forward, front foot ¼ step forward, kamae **(kizami zuki, oi zuki, gyaku zuki, oi zuki, gyaku zuki)***

60) kamae, rear foot ½ step forward jab, front foot ½ step forward reverse punch, rear leg front snap kick, lunge punch to full front stance, rear foot ½ step forward, front foot ¼ step forward reverse punch, rear foot ½ step forward, front foot ¼ step forward, kamae **(kizami zuki, gyaku zuki, gyaku mae geri, oi zuki, gyaku zuki)**

61) kamae, rear foot ½ step forward jab, front foot ½ step forward reverse punch, lunge punch to full front stance, rear foot ½ step forward, same hand jab to full front stance, rear foot ½ step forward, front foot ¼ step forward reverse punch, rear foot ½ step forward, front foot ¼ step forward, kamae **(kizami zuki, gyaku zuki, oi zuki, kizami zuki, gyaku zuki)**

62) kamae, front foot ¼ step forward reverse punch, rear leg front snap kick, same hand lunge punch to full front stance, rear foot ½ step forward, same hand jab to full front stance, rear foot ½ step forward, front foot ¼ step forward reverse punch, rear foot ½ step forward, front foot ¼ step forward, kamae **(gyaku zuki, gyaku mae geri, oi zuki, kizami zuki, gyaku zuki)**

63) kamae, front foot ¼ step forward reverse punch, rear foot full step forward reverse punch, rear leg front snap kick, lunge punch to full front stance, rear foot ½ step forward, front foot ¼ step forward reverse punch, rear foot ½ step forward, front foot ¼ step forward, kamae **(gyaku zuki, gyaku zuki, gyaku mae geri, oi zuki, gyaku zuki)**

64) kamae, lunge punch to full front stance, rear foot ½ step forward, front foot ½ step forward reverse punch, rear leg front snap kick, lunge punch to full front stance, rear foot ½ step forward, front foot ¼ step forward reverse punch, rear foot ½ step forward, front foot ¼ step forward, kamae **(oi zuki, gyaku zuki, gyaku mae geri, oi zuki, gyaku zuki)**

65) kamae, rear leg front snap kick, lunge punch to full front stance, rear foot ½ step forward, front leg snap kick, same hand jab to full front stance, rear foot ½ step forward, front foot ¼ step forward reverse punch, rear foot ½ step forward, front foot ¼ step forward, kamae **(gyaku mae geri, oi zuki, kizami mae geri, kizami zuki, gyaku zuki)**

66) kamae, front leg snap kick, same side jab, reverse punch to full front stance, rear leg front snap kick, lunge punch to full front stance, rear foot ½ step forward, front foot ¼ step forward reverse punch, rear foot ½ step forward, front foot ¼ step forward, kamae **(kizami mae geri, kizami zuki, gyaku zuki, gyaku mae geri, oi zuki, gyaku zuki)**

67) kamae, front foot ¼ step forward reverse punch, rear leg front snap kick, lunge punch to full front stance, rear foot ½ step forward, front leg snap kick, same hand jab to full front stance, rear foot ½ step forward, front foot ¼ step forward reverse punch, rear foot ½ step forward, front foot

¼ step forward, kamae **(gyaku zuki, gyaku mae geri, oi zuki, kizami mae geri, kizami zuki, gyaku zuki)**

Sequential Last Steps

- kamae, front foot ¼ step forward jab, rear foot ½ step forward, front foot ½ step forward reverse punch, rear foot full step forward reverse punch, rear foot ½ step forward, front foot ¼ step forward, kamae (**kizami zuki, gyaku zuki, gyaku zuki**)
- kamae, rear foot ½ step forward jab, front foot ½ step forward reverse punch, rear foot full step forward reverse punch, rear foot ½ step forward, front foot ¼ step forward, kamae (**kizami zuki, gyaku zuki, gyaku zuki**)
- kamae, lunge punch to full front stance, rear foot ½ step forward, front foot ½ step forward reverse punch, rear foot full step forward reverse punch, rear foot ½ step forward, front foot ¼ step forward, kamae (**oi zuki, gyaku zuki, gyaku zuki**)
- kamae, front foot ¼ step forward jab, lunge punch to full front stance, rear foot ½ step forward, front foot ¼ step forward reverse punch, rear foot forward ½ step, front foot ¼ step forward, kamae (**kizami zuki, oi zuki, gyaku zuki**)
- kamae, front foot ¼ step forward reverse punch, same hand lunge punch to full front stance, rear foot ½ step forward, front foot ¼ step forward reverse punch, rear foot ½ step forward, front foot ¼ step forward, kamae (**gyaku zuki, oi zuki, gyaku zuki**)
- kamae, rear foot full step forward reverse punch with front hand, same hand lunge punch to full front stance, rear foot ½ step forward, front foot ¼ step forward reverse punch, rear foot ½ step forward, front foot ¼ step forward, kamae (**kizami gyaku zuki, oi zuki, gyaku zuki**)
- kamae, rear leg front snap kick, lunge punch to full front stance, rear foot ½ step forward, front foot ¼ step forward reverse punch, rear foot ½ step forward, front foot ¼ step forward, kamae (**gyaku mae geri, oi zuki, gyaku zuki**)*
- kamae, front foot ¼ step forward jab, rear foot ½ step forward, front foot ½ step forward reverse punch, rear foot ½ step forward, front foot ¼ step forward, lunge punch to full front stance, rear foot ½ step forward, front foot ½ step forward reverse punch, rear foot ½ step forward, front foot ¼ step forward, kamae (**kizami zuki, gyaku zuki, oi zuki, gyaku zuki**)
- kamae, front foot ¼ step forward jab, rear leg front snap kick, lunge punch to full front stance, rear foot ½ step forward, front foot ¼ step forward, kamae (**kizami zuki, gyaku mae geri, oi zuki, gyaku zuki**)
- kamae, rear foot ½ step forward jab, front foot ½ step forward reverse punch, lunge punch to full front stance, rear foot ½ step forward, front foot ¼ step forward reverse punch, rear foot ½ step forward, front foot ¼ step forward, kamae (**kizami zuki, gyaku zuki, oi zuki, gyaku zuki**)
- kamae, front foot ¼ step forward reverse punch, rear foot full step forward reverse punch, rear foot full step forward lunge punch, rear foot ½ step forward, front foot ¼ step forward reverse punch, rear foot ½ step forward, front foot ¼ step forward, kamae (**gyaku zuki, gyaku zuki, oi zuki, gyaku zuki**)
- kamae, front foot ¼ step forward jab, lunge punch to full front stance, rear foot ½ step forward, front foot ¼ step forward reverse punch, lunge punch to full front stance, rear foot ½ step forward, front foot ¼ step forward reverse punch, rear foot ½ step forward, front foot ¼ step forward, kamae (**kizami zuki, oi zuki, gyaku zuki, oi zuki, gyaku zuki**)*
- kamae, front foot ¼ step forward reverse punch, rear leg front snap kick, lunge punch to full front stance, rear foot ½ step forward, front foot ¼ step forward reverse punch, rear foot ½ step forward, front foot ¼ step forward, kamae (**gyaku zuki, gyaku mae geri, oi zuki, gyaku zuki**)
- kamae, rear foot full step forward reverse punch with front hand, rear leg front snap kick, lung punch with same hand to full stance, rear foot ½ step forward, front foot ¼ step forward reverse punch, rear foot forward ½ step, front foot ¼ step forward, kamae (**kizami gyaku zuki, gyaku mae geri, oi zuki, gyaku zuki**)

168

- kamae, front leg snap kick, kamae, rear leg front snap kick, lunge punch to full front stance, rear foot ½ step forward, front foot ¼ step forward reverse punch, rear foot ½ step forward, front foot ¼ step forward, kamae (**kizami mae geri, gyaku mae geri, oi zuki, gyaku zuki**)
- kamae, rear foot ½ step forward jab, front foot ½ step forward reverse punch, rear leg front snap kick, lunge punch to full front stance, rear foot ½ step forward, front foot ¼ step forward reverse punch, rear foot ½ step forward, front foot ¼ step forward, kamae (**kizami zuki, gyaku zuki, gyaku mae geri, oi zuki, gyaku zuki**)
- kamae, front foot ¼ step forward reverse punch, rear foot full step forward reverse punch, rear leg front snap kick, lunge punch to full front stance, rear foot ½ step forward, front foot ¼ step forward reverse punch, rear foot ½ step forward, front foot ¼ step forward, kamae (**gyaku zuki, gyaku zuki, gyaku mae geri, oi zuki, gyaku zuki**)
- kamae, lunge punch to full front stance, rear foot ½ step forward, front foot ½ step forward reverse punch, rear leg front snap kick, lunge punch to full front stance, rear foot ½ step forward, front foot ¼ step forward reverse punch, rear foot ½ step forward, front foot ¼ step forward, kamae (**oi zuki, gyaku zuki, gyaku mae geri, oi zuki, gyaku zuki**)
- kamae, front leg snap kick, same side jab, reverse punch to full front stance, rear leg front snap kick, lunge punch to full front stance, rear foot ½ step forward, front foot ¼ step forward reverse punch, rear foot ½ step forward, front foot ¼ step forward, kamae (**kizami mae geri, kizami zuki, gyaku zuki, gyaku mae geri, oi zuki, gyaku zuki**)
- kamae, front foot ¼ step forward reverse punch, rear foot ½ step forward jab, front foot ½ step forward reverse punch, rear foot ½ step forward, front foot ¼ step forward, kamae (**gyaku zuki, kizami zuki, gyaku zuki**)*
- kamae, lunge punch to full front stance, rear foot ½ step forward, front foot ¼ step forward same hand jab, rear foot ½ step forward, front foot ¼ step forward reverse punch, rear foot ½ step forward, front foot ¼ step forward, kamae (**oi zuki, kizami zuki, gyaku zuki**)
- kamae, rear foot full step forward reverse punch with front hand, rear foot ½ step forward jab, front foot ¼ step forward reverse punch, rear foot forward ½ step, front foot ¼ step forward, kamae (**kizami gyaku zuki, kizami zuki, gyaku zuki**)
- kamae, front leg snap kick, same side jab, reverse punch to full front stance, front foot back, kamae (**kizami mae geri, kizami zuki, gyaku zuki**)
- kamae, front foot ¼ step forward reverse punch, same hand lunge punch to full front stance, rear foot ½ step forward, same hand jab to full front stance, , rear foot ½ step forward jab, front foot ½ step forward reverse punch rear foot ½ step forward, front foot ¼ step forward, kamae (**gyaku zuki, oi zuki, kizami zuki, gyaku zuki**)
- kamae, rear foot ½ step forward jab, front foot ½ step forward reverse punch, lunge punch to full front stance, rear foot ½ step forward, same hand jab to full front stance, rear foot ½ step forward, front foot ¼ step forward reverse punch, rear foot ½ step forward, front foot ¼ step forward, kamae (**kizami zuki, gyaku zuki, oi zuki, kizami zuki, gyaku zuki**)
- kamae, front foot ¼ step forward reverse punch, rear leg front snap kick, same hand lunge punch to full front stance, rear foot ½ step forward, same hand jab to full front stance, rear foot ½ step forward, front foot ¼ step forward reverse punch, rear foot ½ step forward, front foot ¼ step forward, kamae (**gyaku zuki, gyaku mae geri, oi zuki, kizami zuki, gyaku zuki**)
- kamae, lunge punch to full front stance, rear foot ½ step forward, front leg snap kick, same hand lunge jab to full front stance, rear foot ½ step forward, front foot ¼ step forward reverse punch, rear foot ½ step forward, front foot ¼ step forward, kamae (**oi zuki, kizami mae geri, kizami zuki, gyaku zuki**)
- kamae, rear leg front snap kick, lunge punch to full front stance, rear foot ½ step forward, front leg snap kick, same hand jab to full front stance, rear foot ½ step forward, front foot ¼ step

169

forward reverse punch, rear foot ½ step forward, front foot ¼ step forward, kamae **(gyaku mae geri, oi zuki, kizami mae geri, kizami zuki, gyaku zuki)**

o kamae, front foot ¼ step forward reverse punch, rear leg front snap kick, lunge punch to full front stance, rear foot ½ step forward, front leg snap kick, same hand jab to full front stance, rear foot ½ step forward, front foot ¼ step forward reverse punch, rear foot ½ step forward, front foot ¼ step forward, kamae **(gyaku zuki, gyaku mae geri, oi zuki, kizami mae geri, kizami zuki, gyaku zuki)**

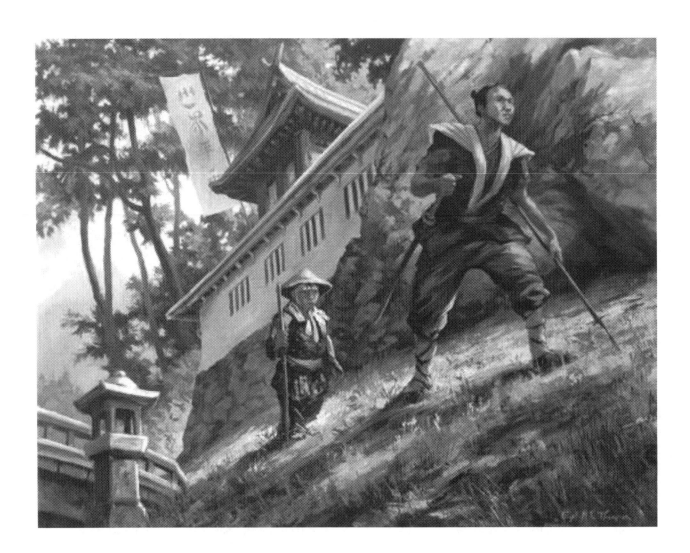

Progressive Groups

- kamae, front foot ¼ step forward jab, rear foot ½ step forward, front foot ¼ step forward, kamae **(kizami zuki)***
- kamae, front foot ¼ step forward jab, rear foot ½ step forward, front foot ½ step forward reverse punch, rear foot ½ step forward, front foot ¼ step forward, kamae **(kizami zuki, gyaku zuki)***
- kamae, front foot ¼ step forward jab, rear foot ½ step forward, front foot ½ step forward reverse punch, rear foot ½ step forward, front foot ¼ step forward, lunge punch to full front stance, rear foot ½ step forward, front foot ½ step forward reverse punch, rear foot ½ step forward, front foot ¼ step forward, kamae **(kizami zuki, gyaku zuki, oi zuki, gyaku zuki)**
- kamae, front foot ¼ step forward jab, lunge punch to full front stance, rear foot ½ step forward, front foot ¼ step forward, kamae **(kizami zuki, oi zuki)***
- kamae, front foot ¼ step forward jab, lunge punch to full front stance, rear foot ½ step forward, front foot ¼ step forward reverse punch, rear foot forward ½ step, front foot ¼ step forward, kamae **(kizami zuki, oi zuki, gyaku zuki)**
- kamae, front foot ¼ step forward jab, lunge punch to full front stance, rear foot ½ step forward, front foot ¼ step forward reverse punch, lunge punch to full front stance, rear foot ½ step forward, front foot ¼ step forward reverse punch, rear foot ½ step forward, front foot ¼ step forward, kamae **(kizami zuki, oi zuki, gyaku zuki, oi zuki, gyaku zuki)***
- kamae, rear foot ½ step forward jab, front foot ½ step forward, kamae **(kizami zuki)**
- kamae, rear foot ½ step forward jab, front foot ½ step forward reverse punch, rear foot ½ step forward, front foot ¼ step forward, kamae **(kizami zuki, gyaku zuki)***
- kamae, rear foot ½ step forward jab, front foot ½ step forward reverse punch, lunge punch to full front stance, rear foot ½ step forward, front foot ¼ step forward reverse punch, rear foot ½ step forward, front foot ¼ step forward, kamae **(kizami zuki, gyaku zuki, oi zuki, gyaku zuki)**
- kamae, front foot ¼ step forward reverse punch, rear foot ½ step forward, front foot ¼ step forward, kamae **(gyaku zuki)***
- kamae, front foot ¼ step forward reverse punch, same hand lunge punch to full front stance, rear foot ½ step forward, front foot ¼ step forward, kamae **(gyaku zuki, oi zuki)**
- kamae, front foot ¼ step forward reverse punch, same hand lunge punch to full front stance, rear foot ½ step forward, front foot ¼ step forward reverse punch, rear foot ½ step forward, front foot ¼ step forward, kamae **(gyaku zuki, oi zuki, gyaku zuki)**
- kamae, front foot ¼ step forward reverse punch, rear foot ½ step forward jab, front foot ¼ step forward, kamae **(gyaku zuki, kizami zuki)**
- kamae, front foot ¼ step forward reverse punch, rear foot ½ step forward jab, front foot ½ step forward reverse punch, rear foot ½ step forward, front foot ¼ step forward, kamae **(gyaku zuki, kizami zuki, gyaku zuki)***
- kamae, front foot ¼ step forward reverse punch, rear leg front snap kick, rear foot ½ step forward, front foot ¼ step forward, kamae **(gyaku zuki, gyaku mae geri)***
- kamae, front foot ¼ step forward reverse punch, rear leg front snap kick, lunge punch to full front stance, rear foot ½ step forward, front foot ¼ step forward reverse punch, rear foot ½ step forward, front foot ¼ step forward, kamae **(gyaku zuki, gyaku mae geri, oi zuki, gyaku zuki)**
- kamae, front foot ¼ step forward reverse punch, rear foot full step forward, kamae **(oi gyaku zuki)***
- kamae, front foot ¼ step forward reverse punch, rear foot full step forward reverse punch, rear foot ½ step forward, front foot ¼ step forward, kamae **(oi gyaku zuki, gyaku zuki)***
- kamae, front foot ¼ step forward reverse punch, rear foot full step forward reverse punch, rear foot full step forward lunge punch, rear foot ½ step forward, front foot ¼ step forward reverse

171

punch, rear foot ½ step forward, front foot ¼ step forward, kamae **(oi gyaku zuki, gyaku zuki, oi zuki, gyaku zuki)**

- o kamae, lunge punch to full front stance, rear foot ½ step forward, front foot ¼ step forward, kamae **(oi zuki)***
- o kamae, lunge punch to full front stance, rear foot ½ step forward, front foot ¼ step forward same hand jab, rear foot ½ step forward, front foot ¼ step forward, kamae **(oi zuki, kizami zuki)***
- o kamae, lunge punch to full front stance, rear foot ½ step forward, front foot ¼ step forward same hand jab, rear foot ½ step forward, front foot ¼ step forward reverse punch, rear foot ½ step forward, front foot ¼ step forward, kamae **(oi zuki, kizami zuki, gyaku zuki)**
- o kamae, lunge punch to full front stance, rear foot ½ step forward, front leg front snap kick to full front stance, rear foot ½ step forward, front foot ¼ step forward, kamae **(oi zuki, kizami mae geri)**
- o kamae, lunge punch to full front stance, rear foot ½ step forward, front leg snap kick, same hand lunge jab to full front stance, rear foot ½ step forward, front foot ¼ step forward reverse punch, rear foot ½ step forward, front foot ¼ step forward, kamae **(oi zuki, kizami mae geri, kizami zuki, gyaku zuki)**
- o kamae, lunge punch to full front stance, rear foot ½ step forward, front foot ¼ step forward reverse punch, rear foot ½ step forward, front foot ¼ step forward, kamae **(oi zuki, gyaku zuki)***
- o kamae, lunge punch to full front stance, rear foot ½ step forward, front foot ½ step forward reverse punch, rear leg front snap kick to full front stance, rear foot ½ step forward, front foot ¼ step forward, kamae **(oi zuki, gyaku zuki, gyaku mae geri)**
- o kamae, lunge punch to full front stance, rear foot ½ step forward, front foot ½ step forward reverse punch, rear leg front snap kick, lunge punch to full front stance, rear foot ½ step forward, front foot ¼ step forward reverse punch, rear foot ½ step forward, front foot ¼ step forward, kamae **(oi zuki, gyaku zuki, gyaku mae geri, oi zuki, gyaku zuki)**
- o kamae, rear foot full step forward reverse punch with front hand, rear foot forward ½ step, front foot ¼ step forward, kamae **(kizami gyaku zuki)**
- o kamae, rear foot full step forward reverse punch with front hand, rear foot ½ step forward jab, front foot ¼ step forward, kamae **(kizami gyaku zuki, kizami zuki)**
- o kamae, rear foot full step forward reverse punch with front hand, rear foot ½ step forward jab, front foot ¼ step forward reverse punch, rear foot forward ½ step, front foot ¼ step forward, kamae **(kizami gyaku zuki, kizami zuki, gyaku zuki)**
- o kamae, rear foot full step forward reverse punch with front hand, same hand lunge punch to full front stance, rear foot ½ step forward, front foot ¼ step forward, kamae **(kizami gyaku zuki, oi zuki)**
- o kamae, rear foot full step forward reverse punch with front hand, same hand lunge punch to full front stance, rear foot ½ step forward, front foot ¼ step forward reverse punch, rear foot ½ step forward, front foot ¼ step forward, kamae **(kizami gyaku zuki, oi zuki, gyaku zuki)**
- o kamae, rear leg front snap kick, lunge punch to full front stance, rear foot ½ step forward, front foot ¼ step forward, kamae **(gyaku mae geri, oi zuki)***
- o kamae, rear leg front snap kick, lunge punch to full front stance, rear foot ½ step forward, front foot ¼ step forward reverse punch, rear foot ½ step forward, front foot ¼ step forward, kamae **(gyaku mae geri, oi zuki, gyaku zuki)***

Unlisted In-Between & Extended Combinations

o kamae, lunge punch to full front stance, reverse punch, rear foot ½ step forward, front foot ¼ step forward, kamae **(oi zuki, gyaku zuki)**

o kamae, rear foot full step forward reverse punch with front hand, same hand lunge punch to full front stance, rear foot ½ step forward, front foot ¼ step forward, kamae **(kizami gyaku zuki, oi zuki)**

o kamae, front foot ¼ step forward jab, rear foot ½ step forward, front foot ¾ step forward reverse punch, rear foot ½ step forward, front foot ¼ step forward, lunge punch to full front stance, rear foot ½ step forward, front foot ¼ step forward, kamae **(kizami zuki, gyaku zuki, oi zuki)**

o kamae, rear foot ½ step forward jab, front foot ¾ step forward reverse punch, lunge punch to full front stance, rear foot ½ step forward, front foot ¼ step forward, kamae **(kizami zuki, gyaku zuki, oi zuki)**

o kamae, front foot ¼ step forward reverse punch, same hand lunge punch to full front stance, rear foot ½ step forward, same hand jab to full front stance, rear foot ½ step forward, front foot ¼ step forward, kamae **(gyaku zuki, oi zuki, kizami zuki)**

o kamae, front foot ¼ step forward reverse punch, rear leg front snap kick, lunge punch to full front stance, rear foot ½ step forward, front foot ¼ step forward, kamae **(gyaku zuki, gyaku mae geri, oi zuki)**

o kamae, front foot ¼ step forward reverse punch, rear foot full step forward reverse punch, rear foot full step forward lunge punch, rear foot ½ step forward, front foot ¼ step forward, kamae **(gyaku zuki, gyaku zuki, oi zuki)**

o kamae, rear foot full step forward reverse punch with front hand, rear leg front snap kick, lung punch with same hand to full stance, rear foot forward ½ step, front foot ¼ step forward, kamae **(kizami gyaku zuki, gyaku mae geri, oi zuki)**

o kamae, front foot ¼ step forward jab, lunge punch to full front stance, rear foot ½ step forward, front foot ¼ step forward reverse punch, lunge punch to full front stance, rear foot ½ step forward, front foot ¼ step forward, kamae **(kizami zuki, oi zuki, gyaku zuki, oi zuki)**

o kamae, rear foot ½ step forward jab, front foot ¾ step forward reverse punch, rear leg front snap kick, lunge punch to full front stance, rear foot ½ step forward, front foot ¼ step forward, kamae **(kizami zuki, gyaku zuki, gyaku mae geri, oi zuki)**

o kamae, front foot ¼ step forward reverse punch, rear foot full step forward reverse punch, rear leg front snap kick, lunge punch to full front stance, rear foot ½ step forward, front foot ¼ step forward, kamae **(gyaku zuki, gyaku zuki, gyaku mae geri, oi zuki)**

o kamae, lunge punch to full front stance, rear foot ½ step forward, front foot ½ step forward reverse punch, rear leg front snap kick, lunge punch to full front stance, rear foot ½ step forward, front foot ¼ step forward, kamae **(oi zuki, gyaku zuki, gyaku mae geri, oi zuki)**

o kamae, front leg snap kick, same side jab, reverse punch to full front stance, rear leg front snap kick, lunge punch to full front stance, rear foot ½ step forward, front foot ¼ step forward, kamae **(kizami mae geri, kizami zuki, gyaku zuki, gyaku mae geri, oi zuki)**

o kamae, front foot ¼ step forward reverse punch, rear leg front snap kick, lunge punch to full front stance, rear foot ½ step forward, front leg snap kick, same hand lunge punch to full front stance, rear foot ½ step forward, front foot ¼ step forward jab, rear foot ½ step forward, front foot ¼ step forward reverse punch, rear foot ½ step forward, front foot ¼ step forward, kamae **(gyaku zuki, gyaku mae geri, oi zuki, kizami mae geri, oi zuki, kizami zuki, gyaku zuki)**

o kamae, front foot ¼ step forward jab then reverse punch, rear leg front snap kick, lunge punch to full front stance, rear foot ½ step forward, front leg snap kick, same hand lunge punch to full front stance, rear foot ½ step forward, front foot ¼ step forward jab, rear foot ½ step forward, front foot ¼ step forward reverse punch, rear foot ½ step forward, front foot ¼ step forward, kamae **(kizami zuki, gyaku zuki, gyaku mae geri, oi zuki, kizami mae geri, oi zuki, kizami zuki, gyaku zuki)**

o   kamae, front leg snap kick, same side jab, reverse punch to full front stance, rear leg front snap kick, lunge punch to full front stance, rear foot ½ step forward, front leg snap kick, same hand jab to full front stance, rear foot ½ step forward, front foot ¼ step forward reverse punch, rear foot ½ step forward, front foot ¼ step forward, kamae **(kizami mae geri, kizami zuki, gyaku zuki, gyaku mae geri, oi zuki, kizami mae geri, kizami zuki, gyaku zuki)**

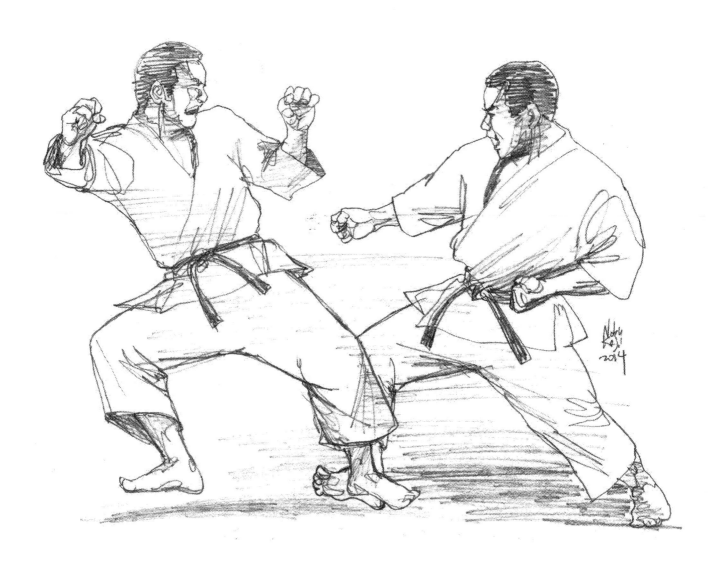

Chapter Fourteen
Combinations with Sweeps

Tsuku Kihon can also be combined with sweeps (ashi-barai) and takedowns. A correctly executed sweep is one of the best ways to disorient an opponent, take him down, and end the fight. There are many types of sweeps: using the bottom of our foot against the ankle (shallow penetration); using the shin against the knee or thigh (medium penetration); using the thigh against the opponent's thigh (deep penetration). Additionally, sweeps can be both inside and outside attacks, the former being the most dangerous and risky, but very devastating to the opponent. Which sweep results depends on the combination used and how close one gets to the other person.

The sweep is highlighted for quick reference in the list of combinations below.

- kamae, rear foot ½ step forward jab, front foot move forward sweep, kamae (**kizami zuki, ashi barai**)
- kamae, rear foot full step forward sweep and jab, kamae (**ashi barai, kizami zuki**)
- kamae, front foot ¼ step forward reverse punch, rear foot ½ step forward, front foot move forward sweep, kamae (**gyaku zuki, ashi barai**)
- kamae, front foot ¼ step forward reverse punch, rear foot full step forward sweep, kamae (**gyaku zuki, ashi barai**)
- kamae, front foot ¼ step forward back fist to full front stance, rear foot ½ step forward, front foot move forward sweep, kamae (**kizami uraken uchi, ashi barai**)
- kamae, lunge punch to full front stance, rear foot ½ step forward, front foot move forward sweep, kamae (**oi zuki, ashi barai**)
- kamae, lunge back fist to full front stance, rear foot ½ step forward, front foot move forward sweep , kamae (**oi uraken uchi, ashi barai**)
- kamae, rear foot full step forward reverse punch with front hand, rear foot forward ½ step, front foot move forward sweep, kamae (**kizami gyaku zuki, ashi barai**)
- kamae, front foot ¼ step forward jab, rear foot ½ step forward, front foot ½ step forward reverse punch, rear foot full move forward sweep, kame (**kizami zuki, gyaku zuki, ashi barai**)
- kamae, front foot ¼ step forward jab, rear foot ½ step forward, front foot move forward sweep, reverse punch, rear foot ½ step forward, front foot ¼ step forward kame (**kizami zuki, ashi barai, gyaku zuki**)
- kamae, front foot ¼ step forward jab, lunge punch to full front stance, rear foot ½ step forward, front foot step forward sweep, kamae (**kizami zuki, oi zuki, ashi barai**)
- kamae, rear foot ½ step forward jab, front foot ½ step forward reverse punch, rear foot full step forward sweep, kamae (**kizami zuki, gyaku zuki, ashi barai**)
- kamae, front foot ¼ step forward reverse punch, same hand lunge punch to full front stance, rear foot ½ step forward, front foot step forward sweep, kamae (**gyaku zuki, oi zuki, ashi barai**)
- kamae, front foot ¼ step forward reverse punch, rear foot full step forward sweep to reverse punch, rear foot ½ step forward, front foot ¼ step forward, kamae (**gyaku zuki, ashi barai, gyaku zuki**)
- kamae, lunge punch to full front stance, rear foot ½ step forward, front foot ¼ step forward reverse punch, rear foot full step forward sweep, kamae (**oi zuki, gyaku zuki, ashi barai**)

- kamae, lunge punch to full front stance, rear foot ½ step forward, front foot move forward sweep to same hand jab, kamae (**oi zuki, ashi barai, kizami zuki**)
- kamae, rear foot full step forward reverse punch with front hand, rear foot ½ step forward jab, front foot move forward sweep, kamae (**kizami gyaku zuki, kizami zuki, ashi barai**)
- kamae, rear foot full step forward reverse punch with front hand, rear foot full step forward sweep to same hand lunge punch, kamae (**kizami gyaku zuki, ashi barai, oi zuki**)
- kamae, rear leg front snap kick lunge punch to full front stance, rear foot ½ step forward, front foot move forward sweep, kamae (**gyaku mae geri, oi zuki, ashi barai**)
- kamae, rear leg round house kick, reverse punch to full front stance, rear foot move forward sweep, kamae (**gyaku mawashi geri, gyaku zuki, ashi barai**)
- kamae, rear leg move forward sweep, same leg round house kick, reverse punch to full front stance, rear foot ½ step forward, front foot ¼ step forward, kamae (**ashi barai, oi mawashi geri, gyaku zuki**)
- kamae, rear leg spinning back kick, reverse punch to full front stance, rear foot move forward sweep, kamae (**uchiro geri, gyaku zuki, ashi barai**)
- kamae, front foot ¼ step forward jab, rear foot ½ step forward, front foot ½ step forward reverse punch, rear foot full step forward sweep to reverse punch, rear foot ½ step forward, front foot ¼ step forward, kamae (**kizami zuki, gyaku zuki, ashi barai, gyaku zuki**)
- kamae, front foot ¼ step forward jab, lunge punch to full front stance, rear foot ½ step forward, front foot move forward sweep to reverse punch, rear foot forward ½ step, front foot ¼ step forward, kamae (**kizami zuki, oi zuki, ashi barai, gyaku zuki**)
- kamae, rear foot ½ step forward jab, front foot ½ step forward reverse punch, rear foot full step forward sweep to reverse punch, rear foot ½ step forward, front foot ¼ step forward, kamae (**kizami zuki, gyaku zuki, ashi barai, gyaku zuki**)
- kamae, front foot ¼ step forward reverse punch, same hand lunge punch to full front stance, rear foot move forward sweep to reverse punch, rear foot ½ step forward, front foot ¼ step forward, kamae (**gyaku zuki, oi zuki, ashi barai, gyaku zuki**)
- kamae, front foot ¼ step forward reverse punch, rear foot ½ step forward jab, front foot move forward sweep to reverse punch, rear foot ½ step forward, front foot ¼ step forward, kamae (**gyaku zuki, kizami zuki, ashi barai, gyaku zuki**)
- kamae, lunge punch to full front stance, rear foot ½ step forward, front foot move forward sweep to same hand jab, rear foot ½ step forward, front foot ¼ step forward reverse punch, rear foot ½ step forward, front foot ¼ step forward, kamae (**oi zuki, ashi barai, kizami zuki, gyaku zuki**)
- kamae, lunge punch to full front stance, rear foot ½ step forward, front foot ½ step forward reverse punch, rear foot full step forward sweep to reverse punch, rear foot ½ step forward, front foot ¼ step forward, kamae (**oi zuki, gyaku zuki, ashi barai, gyaku zuki**)
- kamae, rear foot full step forward reverse punch with front hand, rear foot ½ step forward jab, front foot move forward sweep to reverse punch, rear foot forward ½ step, front foot ¼ step forward, kamae (**kizami gyaku zuki, kizami zuki, ashi barai, gyaku zuki**)
- kamae, rear foot full step forward reverse punch with front hand, rear leg move forward sweep to lunge punch, rear foot ½ step forward, front foot ¼ step forward reverse punch, rear foot ½ step forward, front foot ¼ step forward, kamae (**kizami gyaku zuki, ashi barai, oi zuki, gyaku zuki**)
- kamae, rear leg front snap kick, lunge punch to full front stance, rear foot ½ step forward, front foot move forward sweep to reverse punch, rear foot ½ step forward, front foot ¼ step forward, kamae (**gyaku mae geri, oi zuki, ashi barai, gyaku zuki**)

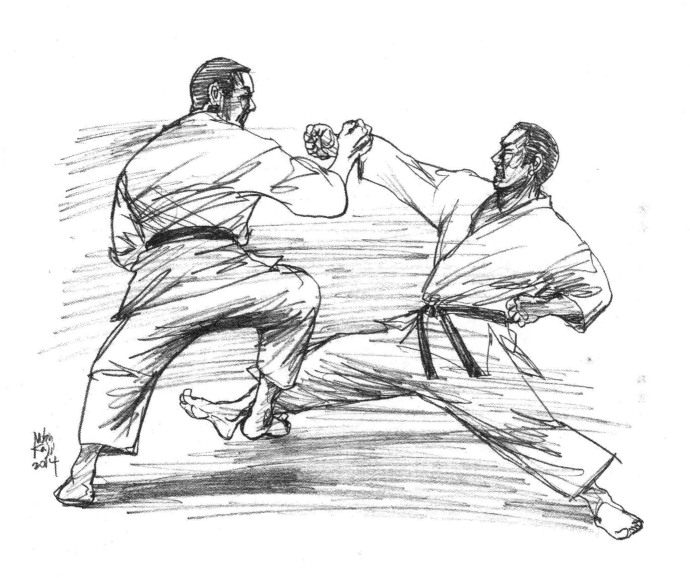

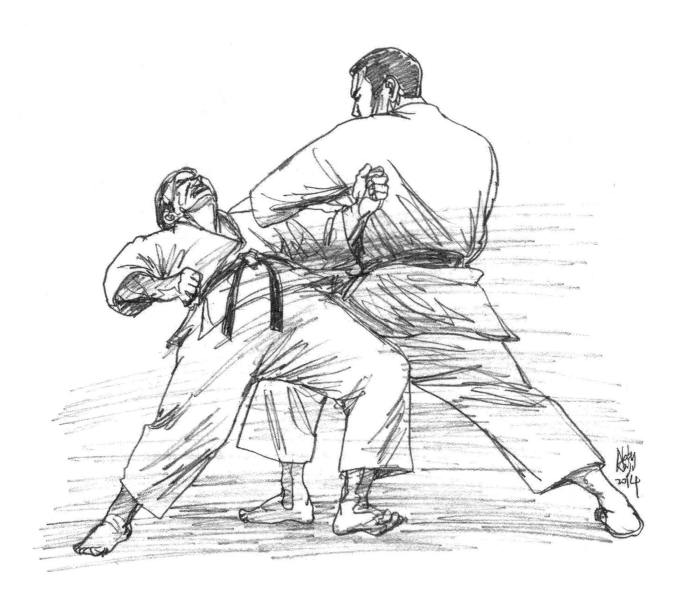

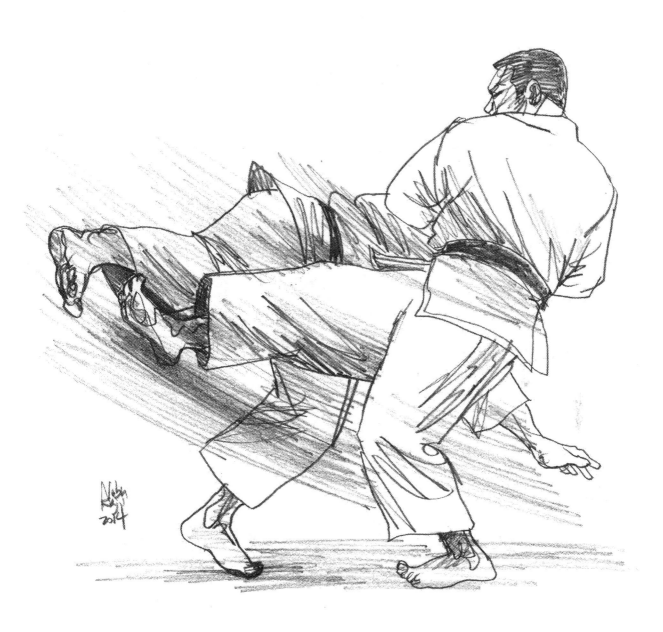

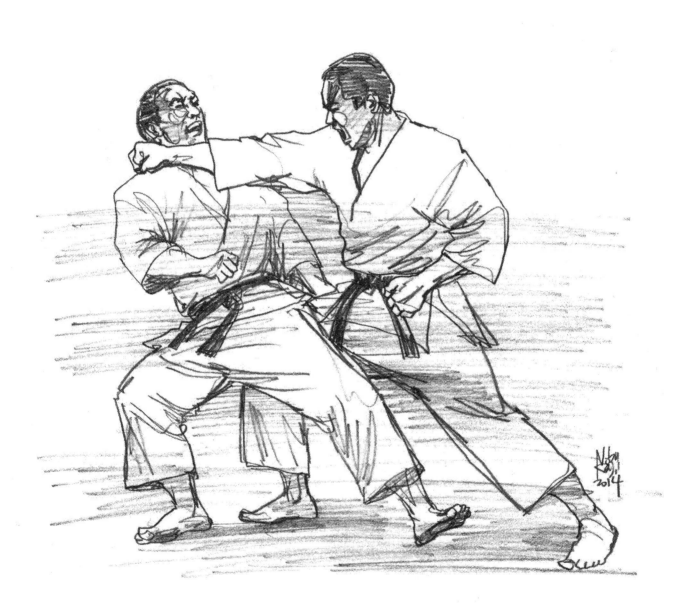

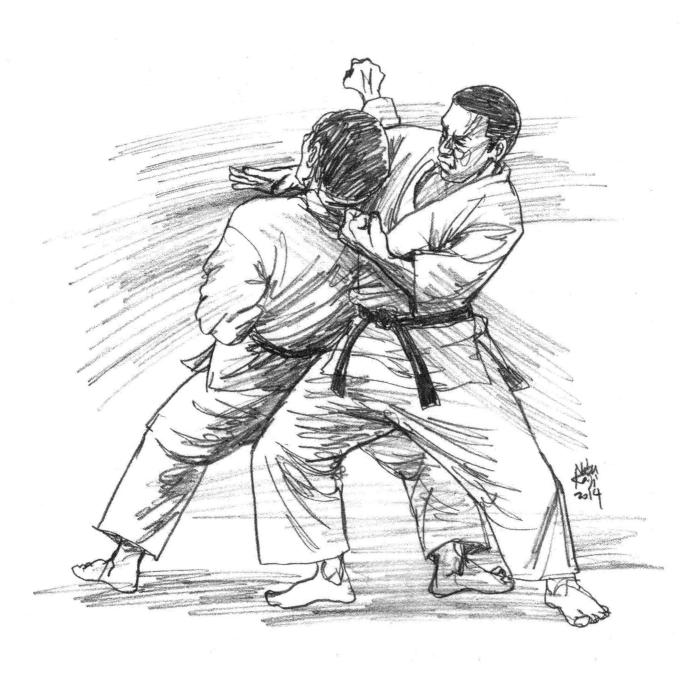

Chapter Fifteen
Belt Level

Tsuku Kihon should be taught starting at brown belt level. However, the most important thing is for the student to have a good grasp of karate kihon and understand body dynamics. Additionally, students starting tusku kihon study must execute correct stances and technique at the point of impact so proper footwork can be developed.

Below is the recommended order and belt level for teaching techniques and combinations.

Brown Belt 1, Sankyu

- kamae, front foot ¼ step forward jab, front foot back, kamae **(kizami zuki)**
- kamae, front foot ¼ step forward reverse punch, front foot back, kamae **(gyaku zuki)**
- kamae, front foot ¼ step forward back fist to full front stance, front foot back, kamae **(kizami uraken uchi)**
- kamae, front foot ¼ step forward jab, reverse punch, bring front foot back, kamae **(kizami zuki, gyaku zuki)**
- kamae, front leg snap kick, same side jab to full front stance, front foot back, kamae **(kizami mae geri, kizami zuki)**
- kamae, front leg snap kick, same side jab, reverse punch to full front stance, front foot back, kamae **(kizami mae geri, kizami zuki, gyaku zuki)**

Brown Belt 2, Nikyu

- kamae, front foot ¼ step forward jab, rear foot ½ step forward, front foot ¼ step forward, kamae **(kizami zuki)**
- kamae, front foot ¼ step forward reverse punch, rear foot ½ step forward, front foot ¼ step forward, kamae **(gyaku zuki)**
- kamae, front foot ¼ step forward reverse punch, rear foot full step forward, kamae **(oi gyaku zuki)**
- kamae, front foot ¼ step forward back fist to full front stance, rear foot ½ step forward, front foot ¼ step forward, kamae **(kizami uraken uchi)**
- kamae, lunge punch to full front stance, rear foot ½ step forward, front foot ¼ step forward, kamae **(oi zuki)**
- kamae, lunge back fist to full front stance, rear foot ½ step forward, front foot ¼ step forward, kamae **(oi uraken uchi)**
- kamae, front foot ¼ step forward jab, rear foot ½ step forward, front foot ½ step forward reverse punch, rear foot ½ step forward, front foot ¼ step forward, kamae **(kizami zuki, gyaku zuki)**
- kamae, rear foot ½ step forward jab, front foot ½ step forward reverse punch, rear foot ½ step forward, front foot ¼ step forward, kamae **(kizami zuki, gyaku zuki)**

- kamae, front foot ¼ step forward reverse punch, rear leg front snap kick, rear foot ½ step forward, front foot ¼ step forward, kamae **(gyaku zuki, gyaku mae geri)**
- kamae, rear leg front snap kick, lunge punch to full front stance, rear foot ½ step forward, front foot ¼ step forward, kamae **(gyaku mae geri, oi zuki)**
- kamae, rear leg front snap kick, lunge back fist to full front stance, rear foot ½ step forward, front foot ¼ step forward, kamae **(gyaku mae geri, oi uraken uchi)**

Brown Belt 3, Ikkyu

- kamae, front foot ¼ step forward jab, rear foot ½ step forward, front foot ¼ step forward, kamae **(kizami zuki)**
- kamae, rear foot ½ step forward jab, front foot ½ step forward, kamae **(kizami zuki)**
- kamae, rear foot full step forward reverse punch with front hand, rear foot forward ½ step, front foot ¼ step forward, kamae **(kizami gyaku zuki)**
- kamae, rear foot ½ step forward jab, rear foot ½ step back reverse punch, kamae **(kizami zuki, gyaku zuki)**
- kamae, front foot ¼ step forward jab, lunge punch to full front stance, rear foot ½ step forward, front foot ¼ step forward, kamae **(kizami zuki, oi zuki)**
- kamae, rear foot ½ step forward reverse punch, rear foot ½ step back jab, kamae **(gyaku zuki, kizami zuki)**
- kamae, front foot ¼ step forward reverse punch, same hand lunge back fist to full front stance, rear foot ½ step forward, front foot ¼ step forward, kamae **(gyaku zuki, oi uraken uchi)**
- kamae, front foot ¼ step forward reverse punch, same hand lunge punch to full front stance, rear foot ½ step forward, front foot ¼ step forward, kamae **(gyaku zuki, oi zuki)**
- kamae, front foot ¼ step forward reverse punch, rear foot ½ step forward jab, front foot ¼ step forward, kamae **(gyaku zuki, kizami zuki)**
- kamae, front foot ¼ step forward reverse punch, rear foot full step forward reverse punch, rear foot ½ step forward, front foot ¼ step forward, kamae **(gyaku zuki, gyaku zuki)**
- kamae, lunge punch to full front stance, rear foot ½ step forward, front foot ¼ step forward same hand back fist, kamae **(oi zuki, oi uraken uchi)**
- kamae, lunge punch to full front stance, rear foot ½ step forward, front foot ¼ step forward reverse punch, rear foot ½ step forward, front foot ¼ step forward, kamae **(oi zuki, gyaku zuki)**
- kamae, lunge punch to full front stance, rear foot ½ step forward, front foot ¼ step forward same hand jab, rear foot ½ step forward, front foot ¼ step forward, kamae **(oi zuki, kizami zuki)**
- kamae, front foot ¼ step forward jab, rear foot ½ step forward, front foot ½ step forward reverse punch, rear foot full step forward reverse punch, rear foot ½ step forward, front foot ¼ step forward, kamae **(kizami zuki, gyaku zuki, gyaku zuki)**
- kamae, front foot ¼ step forward reverse punch, same hand lunge punch to full front stance, rear foot ½ step forward, front foot ¼ step forward reverse punch, rear foot ½ step forward, front foot ¼ step forward, kamae **(gyaku zuki, oi zuki, gyaku zuki)**
- kamae, lunge punch to full front stance, rear foot ½ step forward, front foot ½ step forward reverse punch, rear foot full step forward reverse punch, rear foot ½ step forward, front foot ¼ step forward, kamae **(oi zuki, gyaku zuki, gyaku zuki)**

- kamae, lunge punch to full front stance, rear foot ½ step forward, front foot ½ step forward reverse punch, rear leg front snap kick to full front stance, rear foot ½ step forward, front foot ¼ step forward, kamae **(oi zuki, gyaku zuki, gyaku mae geri)**
- kamae, rear leg front snap kick, lunge punch to full front stance, rear foot ½ step forward, front foot ¼ step forward reverse punch, rear foot ½ step forward, front foot ¼ step forward, kamae **(gyaku mae geri, oi zuki, gyaku zuki)**
- kamae, front foot ¼ step forward jab, rear foot ½ step forward, front foot ½ step forward reverse punch, rear foot ½ step forward, front foot ¼ step forward, lunge punch to full front stance, rear foot ½ step forward, front foot ½ step forward reverse punch, rear foot ½ step forward, front foot ¼ step forward, kamae **(kizami zuki, gyaku zuki, oi zuki, gyaku zuki)**
- kamae, front foot ¼ step forward reverse punch, rear leg front snap kick, lunge punch to full front stance, rear foot ½ step forward, front foot ¼ step forward reverse punch, rear foot ½ step forward, front foot ¼ step forward, kamae **(gyaku zuki, gyaku mae geri, oi zuki, gyaku zuki)**
- kamae, front foot ¼ step forward reverse punch, rear foot full step forward reverse punch, rear foot full step forward lunge punch, rear foot ½ step forward, front foot ¼ step forward reverse punch, rear foot ½ step forward, front foot ¼ step forward, kamae **(gyaku zuki, gyaku zuki, oi zuki, gyaku zuki)**
- kamae, front foot ¼ step forward jab, lunge punch to full front stance, rear foot ½ step forward, front foot ¼ step forward reverse punch, lunge punch to full front stance, rear foot ½ step forward, front foot ¼ step forward reverse punch, rear foot ½ step forward, front foot ¼ step forward, kamae **(kizami zuki, oi zuki, gyaku zuki, oi zuki, gyaku zuki)**

First Degree Black Belt, Shodan

- kamae, rear leg round house kick, reverse punch to full front stance, rear foot ½ step forward, front foot ¼ step forward, kamae **(gyaku mawashi geri, gyaku zuki)**
- kamae, rear leg side thrust kick, lunge back fist to full front stance, rear foot ½ step forward, front foot ¼ step forward, kamae **(gyaku yoko geri, oi uraken uchi)**
- kamae, rear leg spinning back kick, reverse punch to full front stance, rear foot ½ step forward, front foot ¼ step forward, kamae **(uchiro geri, gyaku zuki)**
- kamae, front foot ¼ step forward jab, lunge punch to full front stance, rear foot ½ step forward, front foot ¼ step forward reverse punch, rear foot forward ½ step, front foot ¼ step forward, kamae **(kizami zuki, oi zuki, gyaku zuki)**
- kamae, rear foot ½ step forward jab, front foot ½ step forward reverse punch, rear foot full step forward reverse punch, rear foot ½ step forward, front foot ¼ step forward, kamae **(kizami zuki, gyaku zuki, gyaku zuki)**
- kamae, front foot ¼ step forward reverse punch, rear foot ½ step forward jab, front foot ½ step forward reverse punch, rear foot ½ step forward, front foot ¼ step forward, kamae **(gyaku zuki, kizami zuki, gyaku zuki)**
- kamae, front leg snap kick, kamae, rear leg round house kick, reverse punch to full front stance, rear foot ½ step forward, front foot ¼ step forward, kamae **(kizami mae geri, gyaku mawashi geri, gyaku zuki)**
- kamae, rear foot ½ step forward jab, front foot ½ step forward reverse punch, lunge punch to full front stance, rear foot ½ step forward, front foot ¼ step forward reverse punch, rear foot

½ step forward, front foot ¼ step forward, kamae **(kizami zuki, gyaku zuki, oi zuki, gyaku zuki)**

- kamae, front leg snap kick, kamae, rear leg front snap kick, lunge punch to full front stance, rear foot ½ step forward, front foot ¼ step forward reverse punch, rear foot ½ step forward, front foot ¼ step forward, kamae **(kizami mae geri, gyaku mae geri, oi zuki, gyaku zuki)**
- kamae, front foot ¼ step forward reverse punch, rear leg front snap kick, same hand lunge punch to full front stance, rear foot ½ step forward, same hand jab to full front stance, rear foot ½ step forward, front foot ¼ step forward reverse punch, rear foot ½ step forward, front foot ¼ step forward, kamae **(gyaku zuki, gyaku mae geri, oi zuki, kizami zuki, gyaku zuki)**

Second Degree Black Belt, Nidan

- kamae, lunge punch to full front stance, rear foot ½ step forward, front leg front snap kick to full front stance, rear foot ½ step forward, front foot ¼ step forward, kamae **(oi zuki, kizami mae geri)**
- kamae, rear foot full step forward reverse punch with front hand, rear foot ½ step forward jab, front foot ¼ step forward, kamae **(kizami gyaku zuki, kizami zuki)**
- kamae, rear foot full step forward reverse punch with front hand, same hand lunge punch to full front stance, rear foot ½ step forward, front foot ¼ step forward, kamae **(kizami gyaku zuki, oi zuki)**
- kamae, lunge punch to full front stance, rear foot ½ step forward, front foot ¼ step forward same hand jab, rear foot ½ step forward, front foot ¼ step forward reverse punch, rear foot ½ step forward, front foot ¼ step forward, kamae **(oi zuki, kizami zuki, gyaku zuki)**
- kamae, rear foot full step forward reverse punch with front hand, rear foot ½ step forward jab, front foot ¼ step forward reverse punch, rear foot forward ½ step, front foot ¼ step forward, kamae **(kizami gyaku zuki, kizami zuki, gyaku zuki)**
- kamae, rear foot full step forward reverse punch with front hand, same hand lunge punch to full front stance, rear foot ½ step forward, front foot ¼ step forward reverse punch, rear foot ½ step forward, front foot ¼ step forward, kamae **(kizami gyaku zuki, oi zuki, gyaku zuki)**
- kamae, rear foot full step forward reverse punch with front hand, rear leg round house kick, reverse punch with same hand to full stance, rear foot forward ½ step, front foot ¼ step forward, kamae **(kizami gyaku zuki, gyaku mawashi geri, gyaku zuki)**
- kamae, front foot ¼ step forward jab, rear leg front snap kick, lunge punch to full front stance, rear foot ½ step forward, front foot ¼ step forward, kamae **(kizami zuki, gyaku mae geri, oi zuki, gyaku zuki)**
- kamae, front foot ¼ step forward reverse punch, same hand lunge punch to full front stance, rear foot ½ step forward, same hand jab to full front stance, rear foot ½ step forward jab, front foot ½ step forward reverse punch rear foot ½ step forward, front foot ¼ step forward, kamae **(gyaku zuki, oi zuki, kizami zuki, gyaku zuki)**
- kamae, lunge punch to full front stance, rear foot ½ step forward, front leg snap kick, same hand lunge jab to full front stance, rear foot ½ step forward, front foot ¼ step forward reverse punch, rear foot ½ step forward, front foot ¼ step forward, kamae **(oi zuki, kizami mae geri, kizami zuki, gyaku zuki)**
- kamae, rear foot full step forward reverse punch with front hand, rear leg front snap kick, lung punch with same hand to full stance, rear foot ½ step forward, front foot ¼ step forward

188

reverse punch, rear foot forward ½ step, front foot ¼ step forward, kamae **(kizami gyaku zuki, gyaku mae geri, oi zuki, gyaku zuki)**

- kamae, rear foot ½ step forward jab, front foot ½ step forward reverse punch, rear leg front snap kick, lunge punch to full front stance, rear foot ½ step forward, front foot ¼ step forward reverse punch, rear foot ½ step forward, front foot step forward, kamae **(kizami zuki, gyaku zuki, gyaku mae geri, oi zuki, gyaku zuki)**
- kamae, rear foot ½ step forward jab, front foot ½ step forward reverse punch, lunge punch to full front stance, rear foot ½ step forward, same hand jab to full front stance, rear foot ½ step forward, front foot ¼ step forward reverse punch, rear foot ½ step forward, front foot ¼ step forward, kamae **(kizami zuki, gyaku zuki, oi zuki, kizami zuki, gyaku zuki)**
- kamae, front foot ¼ step forward reverse punch, rear foot full step forward reverse punch, rear leg front snap kick, lunge punch to full front stance, rear foot ½ step forward, front foot ¼ step forward reverse punch, rear foot ½ step forward, front foot ¼ step forward, kamae **(gyaku zuki, gyaku zuki, gyaku mae geri, oi zuki, gyaku zuki)**
- kamae, lunge punch to full front stance, rear foot ½ step forward, front foot ½ step forward reverse punch, rear leg front snap kick, lunge punch to full front stance, rear foot ½ step forward, front foot ¼ step forward reverse punch, rear foot ½ step forward, front foot ¼ step forward, kamae **(oi zuki, gyaku zuki, gyaku mae geri, oi zuki, gyaku zuki)**

Third Degree Black Belt, Sandan

- kamae, rear leg front snap kick, lunge punch to full front stance, rear foot ½ step forward, front leg snap kick, same hand jab to full front stance, rear foot ½ step forward, front foot ¼ step forward reverse punch, rear foot ½ step forward, front foot ¼ step forward, kamae **(gyaku mae geri, oi zuki, kizami mae geri, kizami zuki, gyaku zuki)**
- kamae, front leg snap kick, same side jab, reverse punch to full front stance, rear leg front snap kick, lunge punch to full front stance, rear foot ½ step forward, front foot ¼ step forward reverse punch, rear foot ½ step forward, front foot ¼ step forward, kamae **(kizami mae geri, kizami zuki, gyaku zuki, gyaku mae geri, oi zuki, gyaku zuki)**
- kamae, front foot ¼ step forward reverse punch, rear leg front snap kick, lunge punch to full front stance, rear foot ½ step forward, front leg snap kick, same hand jab to full front stance, rear foot ½ step forward, front foot ¼ step forward reverse punch, rear foot ½ step forward, front foot ¼ step forward, kamae **(gyaku zuki, gyaku mae geri, oi zuki, kizami mae geri, kizami zuki, gyaku zuki)**

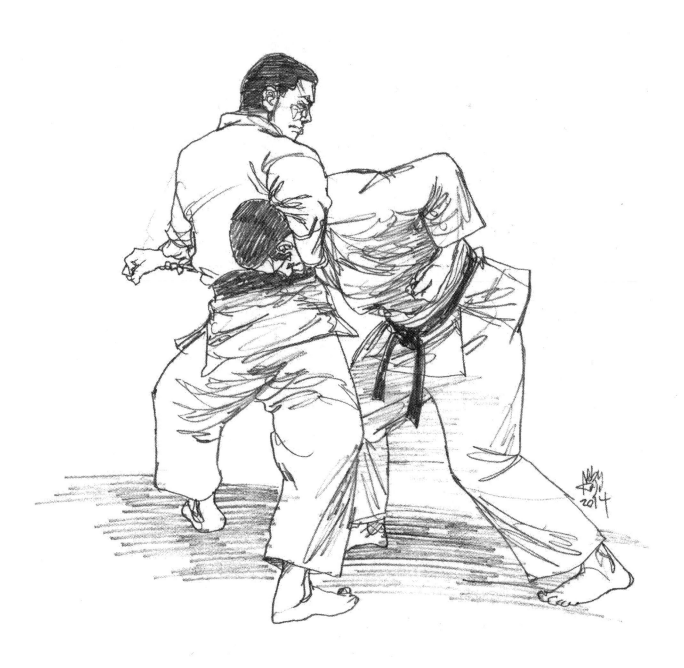

Appendix

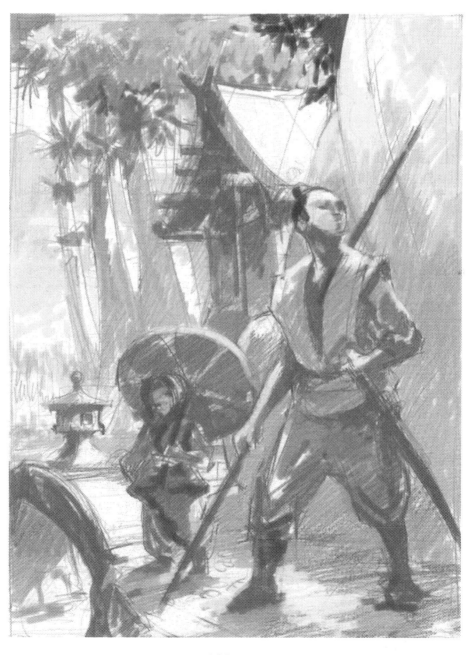

191

Lineage – Shinkyu Shotokan Karate

Below are the original 25 Tsuku Kihon combinations taught by sensei Leroy Rodrigues at the Shinkyu Shotokan Karate dojo. They are all marked by an asterisk throughout this book to indicate origin.

- kamae, front foot ¼ step forward jab, front foot back, kamae **(kizami zuki)***
- kamae, front foot ¼ step forward jab, rear foot ½ step forward, front foot ¼ step forward, kamae **(kizami zuki)***
- kamae, rear foot ½ step forward jab, rear foot ½ step back, kamae **(kizami zuki)***
- kamae, rear foot ½ step forward jab, front foot ½ step forward, kamae **(kizami zuki)***
- kamae, front foot ¼ step forward reverse punch, front foot back, kamae **(gyaku zuki)***
- kamae, front foot ¼ step forward reverse punch, rear foot ½ step forward, front foot ¼ step forward, kamae **(gyaku zuki)***
- kamae, front foot ¼ step forward reverse punch, rear foot full step forward, kamae **(oi gyaku zuki)***
- kamae, lunge punch to full front stance, rear foot ½ step forward, front foot ¼ step forward, kamae **(oi zuki)***
- kamae, lunge back fist to full front stance, rear foot ½ step forward, front foot ¼ step forward, kamae **(oi uraken uchi)***
- kamae, front foot ¼ step forward jab, rear foot ½ step forward, front foot ½ step forward reverse punch, rear foot ½ step forward, front foot ¼ step forward, kamae **(kizami zuki, gyaku zuki)***
- kamae, front foot ¼ step forward jab, lunge punch to full front stance, rear foot ½ step forward, front foot ¼ step forward, kamae **(kizami zuki, oi zuki)***
- kamae, front foot ¼ step forward reverse punch, same hand lunge back fist to full front stance, rear foot ½ step forward, front foot ¼ step forward, kamae **(gyaku zuki, oi uraken uchi)***
- kamae, front foot ¼ step forward reverse punch, rear leg front snap kick, rear foot ½ step forward, front foot ¼ step forward, kamae **(gyaku zuki, gyaku mae geri)***
- kamae, front foot ¼ step forward reverse punch, rear foot full step forward reverse punch, rear foot ½ step forward, front foot ¼ step forward, kamae **(gyaku zuki, gyaku zuki)***
- kamae, lunge punch to full front stance, rear foot ½ step forward, front foot ¼ step forward same hand back fist, kamae **(oi zuki, oi uraken uchi)***
- kamae, lunge punch to full front stance, rear foot ½ step forward, front foot ¼ step forward reverse punch, rear foot ½ step forward, front foot ¼ step forward, kamae **(oi zuki, gyaku zuki)***
- kamae, lunge punch to full front stance, rear foot ½ step forward, front foot ¼ step forward same hand jab, rear foot ½ step forward, front foot ¼ step forward, kamae **(oi zuki, kizami zuki)***
- kamae, rear leg round house kick, reverse punch to full front stance, rear foot ½ step forward, front foot ¼ step forward, kamae **(gyaku mawashi geri, gyaku zuki)***
- kamae, rear leg side thrust kick, lunge back fist to full front stance, rear foot ½ step forward, front foot ¼ step forward, kamae **(gyaku yoko geri, oi uraken uchi)***
- kamae, rear leg spinning back kick, reverse punch to full front stance, rear foot ½ step forward, front foot ¼ step forward, kamae **(uchiro geri, gyaku zuki)***
- kamae, rear leg front snap kick, lunge back fist to full front stance, rear foot ½ step forward, front foot ¼ step forward, kamae **(gyaku mae geri, oi uraken uchi)***
- kamae, rear leg front snap kick, lunge punch to full front stance, rear foot ½ step forward, front foot ¼ step forward, kamae **(gyaku mae geri, oi zuki)***

- kamae, front foot ¼ step forward reverse punch, rear foot ½ step forward jab, front foot ½ step forward reverse punch, rear foot ½ step forward, front foot ¼ step forward, kamae **(gyaku zuki, kizami zuki, gyaku zuki)***
- kamae, rear leg front snap kick, lunge punch to full front stance, rear foot ½ step forward, front foot ¼ step forward reverse punch, rear foot ½ step forward, front foot ¼ step forward, kamae **(gyaku mae geri, oi zuki, gyaku zuki)***
- kamae, front foot ¼ step forward jab, lunge punch to full front stance, rear foot ½ step forward, front foot ¼ step forward reverse punch, lunge punch to full front stance, rear foot ½ step forward, front foot ¼ step forward reverse punch, rear foot ½ step forward, front foot ¼ step forward, kamae **(kizami zuki, oi zuki, gyaku zuki, oi zuki, gyaku zuki)***

Select Bibliography

Shigeru Egami, *The Heart of Karate-Do* (1976, Tokyo).

Keinosuke Enoeda, *Shotokan Karate: 5th Kyu to Black Belt* (1996, London).

Emil Farcas & John Corcoran, *The Overlook Martial Arts Dictionary* (1983, New York).

Jose M. Fraguas, *Karate Masters* (Burbank, 2001).

Gichin Funakoshi, translated by Tsutomu Ohshima, *Karate-Do Kyohan: The Master Text* (New York, 1973).

Hirokazu Kanazawa, *Shotokan Karate International Kata Vol.1* (1981, Tokyo).

Hirokazu Kanazawa, *Shotokan Karate International Kata Vol.2* (1982, Tokyo).

Hirokazu Kanazawa, *The Complete Kumite: Karate Fighting Techniques* (2004, Tokyo).

Richard 'Biggie' Kim, *The Weaponless Warriors: An Informal History of Okinawan Karate* (1974, Burbank).

Richard 'Biggie' Kim, *The Classical Man* (1982, Canada).

Steve McCann & Bernardo Mercado, *Karate Everyone, 2nd Edition* (2012, Winston-Salem).

Masatoshi Nakayama, *Practical Karate Series* (1963, Tokyo).

Masatoshi Nakayama, *Dynamic Karate* (1966, Tokyo).

Masatoshi Nakayama, *Best Karate Series* (1977, Tokyo).

Hidetaka Nishiyama & Richard C. Brown, *Karate: The Art of "Empty Hand" Fighting* (Tokyo, 1959).

Masutatsu Oyama, *Vital Karate* (1967, San Francisco).

Mas Oyama, *Essential Karate* (1975, Tokyo).

Masutatsu Oyama, *Mastering Karate* (1966, New York).

Mayer H. Parry, *A Basic Glossary of Bujutsu* (1975, Scotland).

Leroy Rodrigues, *Classic Kata of Shorinji Ryu: Okinawan Karate Forms of Richard 'Biggie' Kim* (2014, Bloomington).

Elmar T. Schmeisser, Ph.D., *Advanced Karate-Do: Concepts, Techniques and Training Methods* (1994, Missouri).

John Sell, Unante: *The Secrets of Karate* (1995, Hollywood).

Shojiro Sugiyama, *25 Shotokan Kata* (1984, Chicago).

Shojiro Sugiyama, *11 Innovations in Karate* (2005, Chicago).

Shojiro Sugiyama, *Kitoh Karate* (1994, Chicago).

Shojiro Sugiyama, *Basic Principles of Karate* (1991, Chicago).

Shojiro Sugiyama, *Kumite-Gata* (1992, Chicago).

Peter Urban, *The Karate Dojo* (1967, Rutland).

Select Filmography

Kuro Obi

Enter the Dragon

The Seven Samurai

Warrior

Ip Man

1st Legends Championships

Choke - Rickson Gracie

Karate: The Art of Empty Hand Fighting - Rising Sun Productions

Shotokan Karate Series – Masatoshi Nakayama

The Art of Combative Motion – Troy Price

Okinawa Makiwaras – Takemi Takayasu

Winning Competition Karate – Yukiyoshi Murutani & Hideharu Igaki

Shotokan Raw Power – Tsunami Productions

Tanaka: The Master – Tsunami Productions

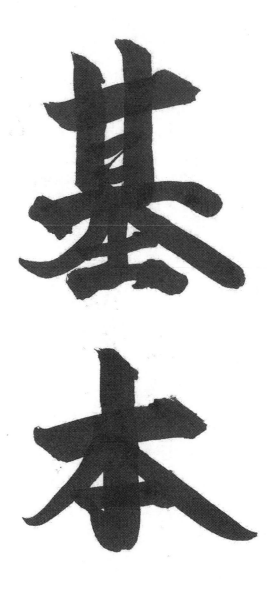

Kihon

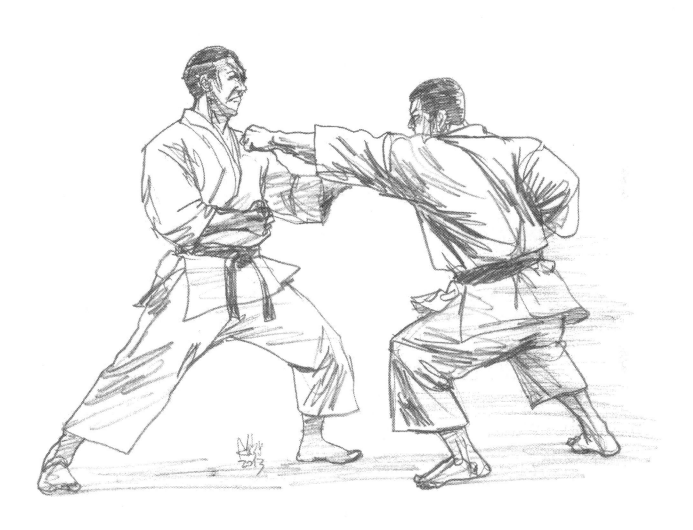

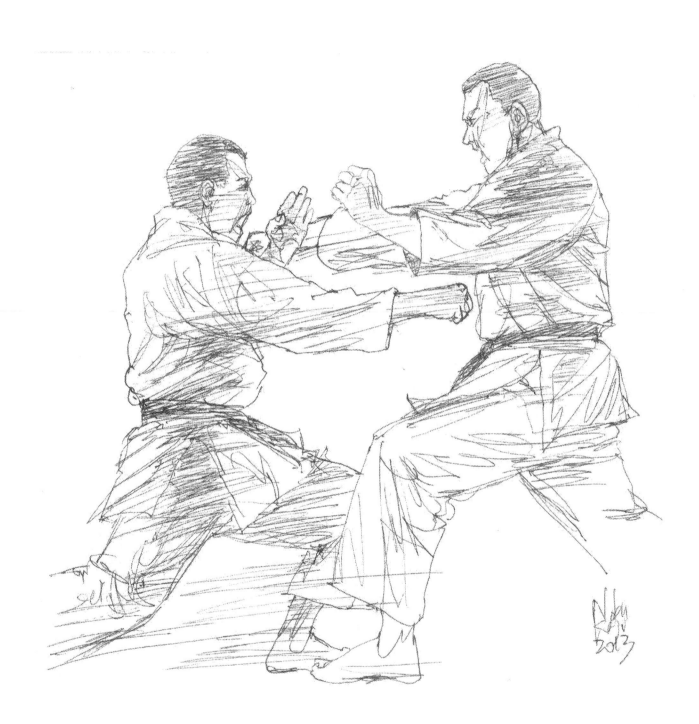

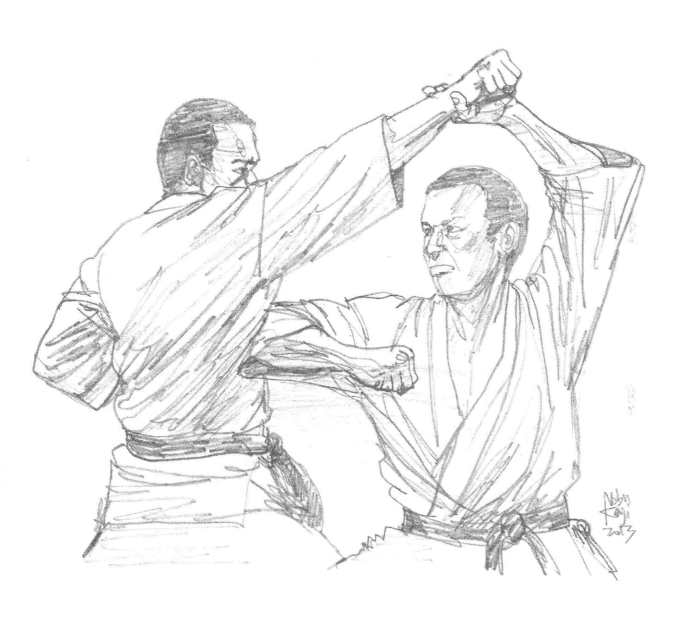

199

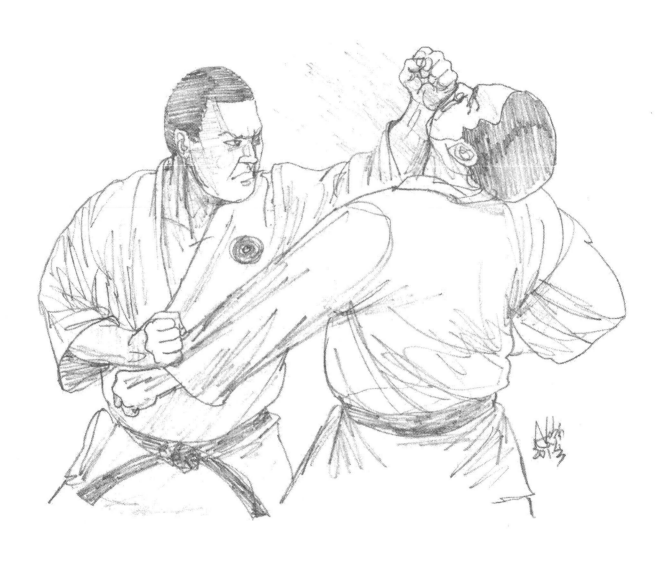

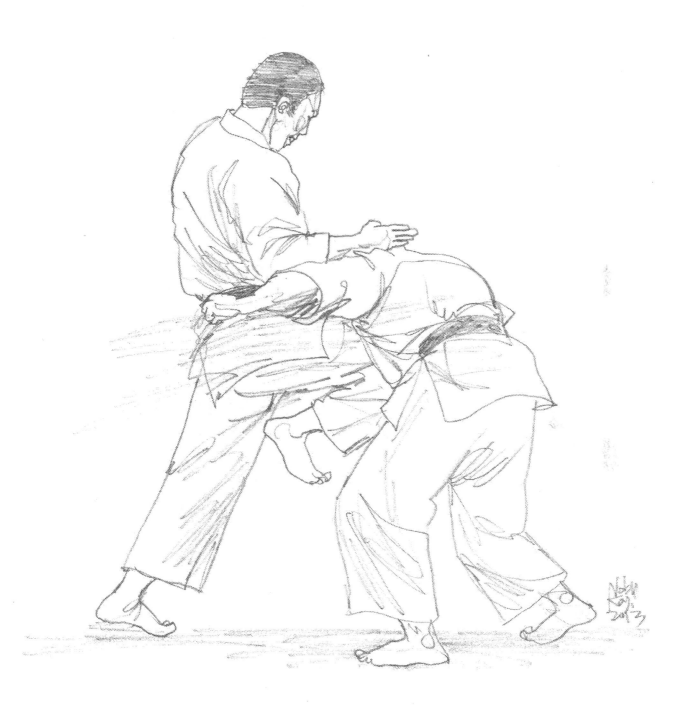

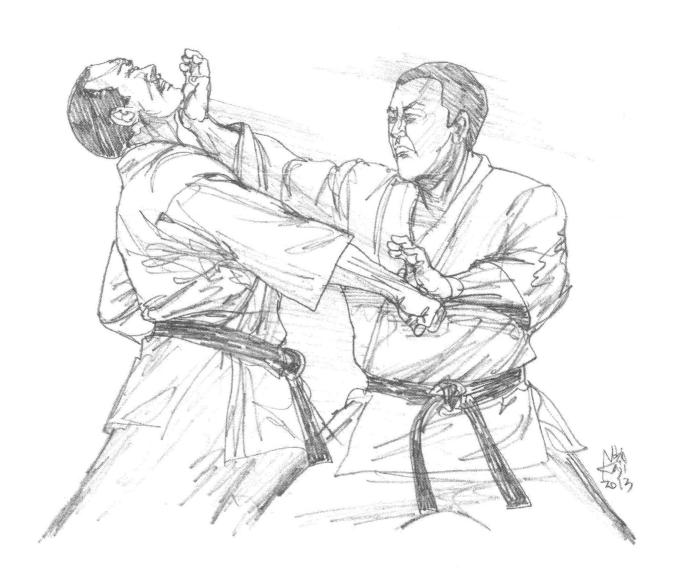

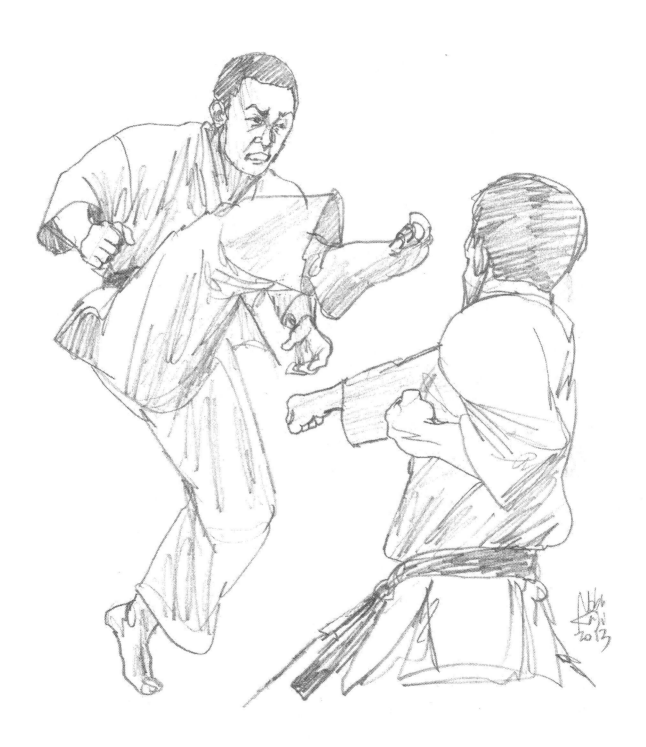

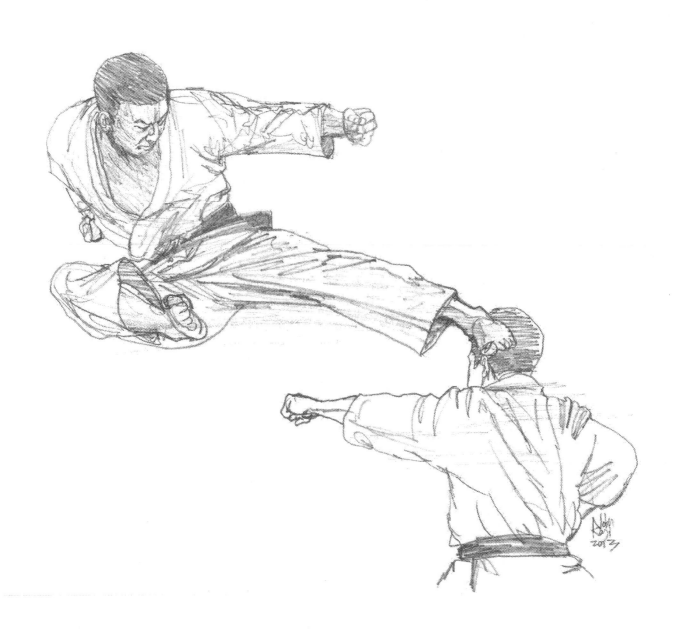

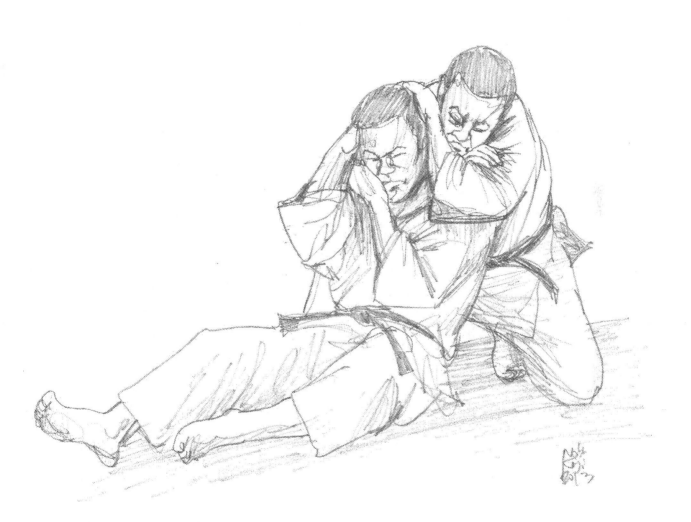

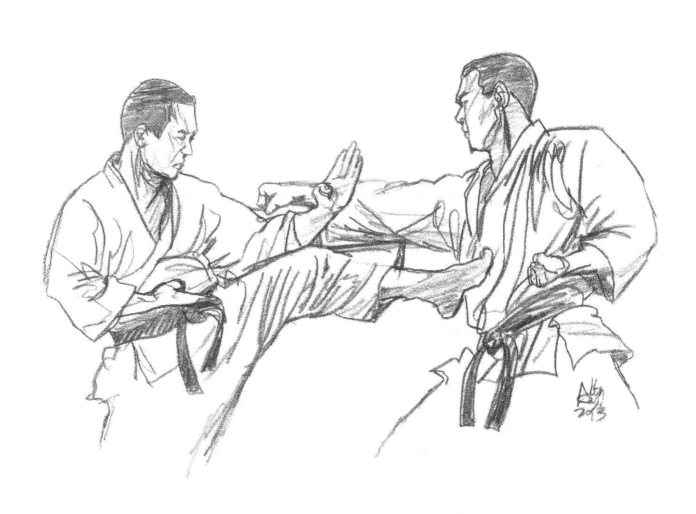

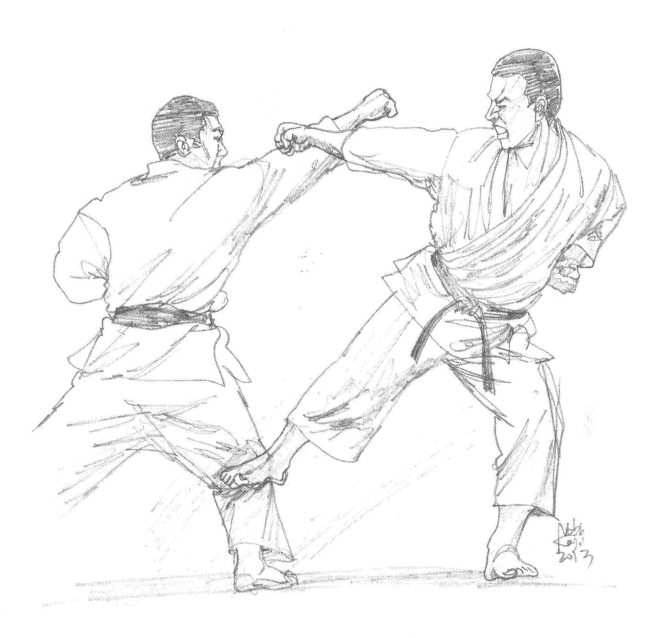

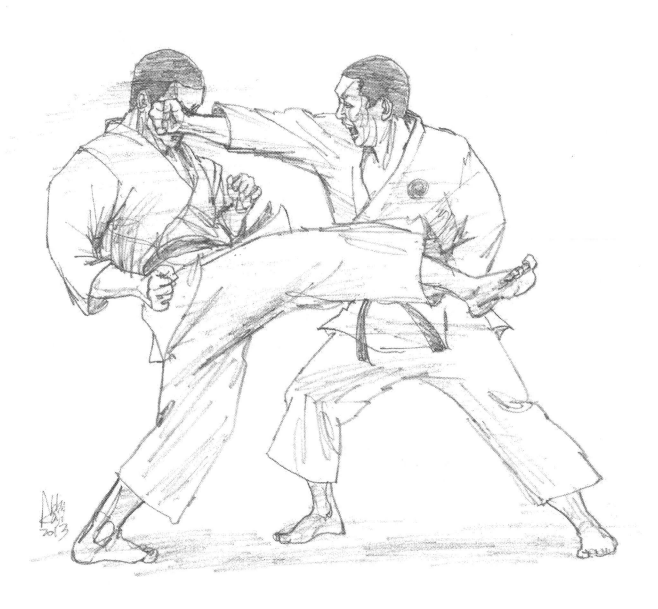

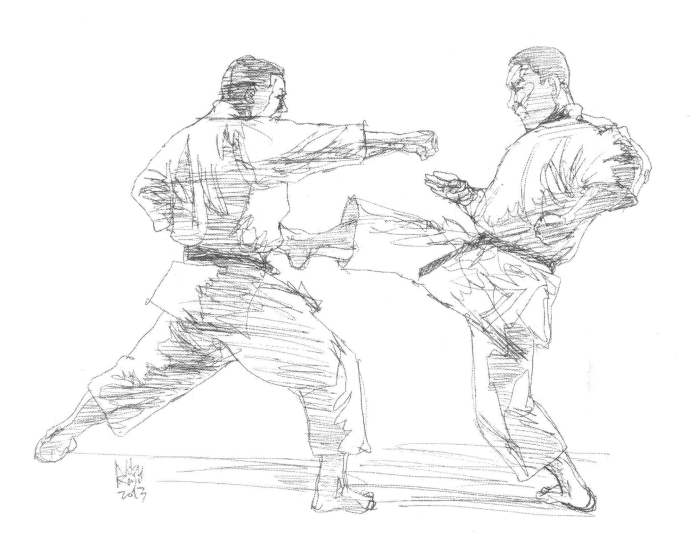

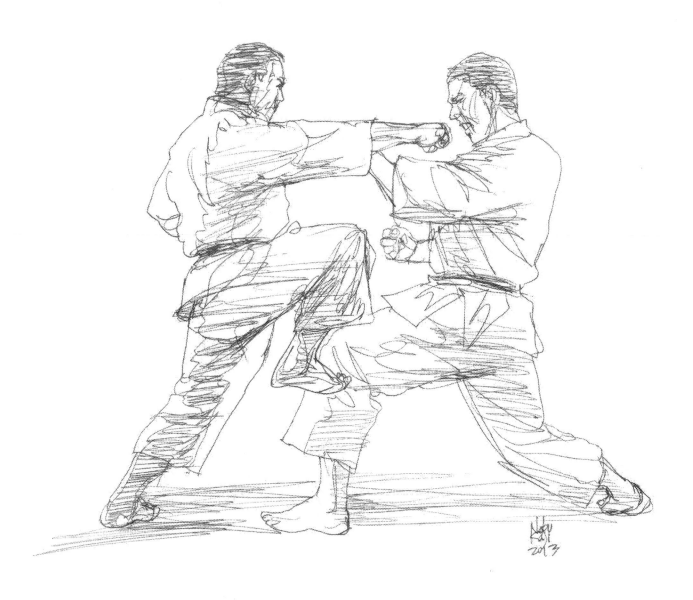

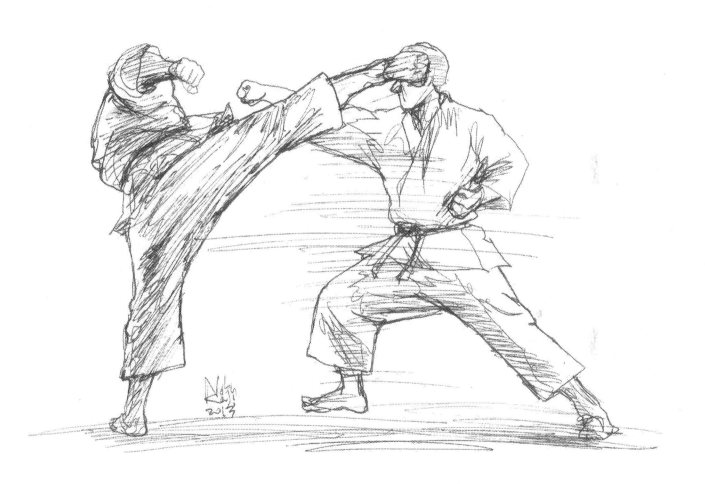

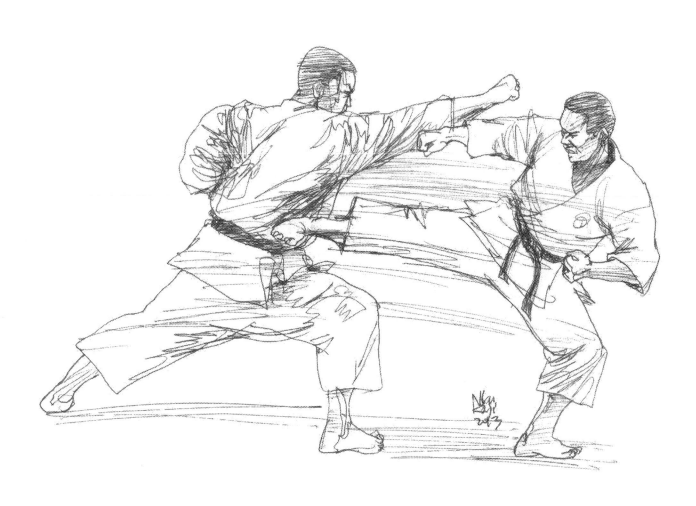

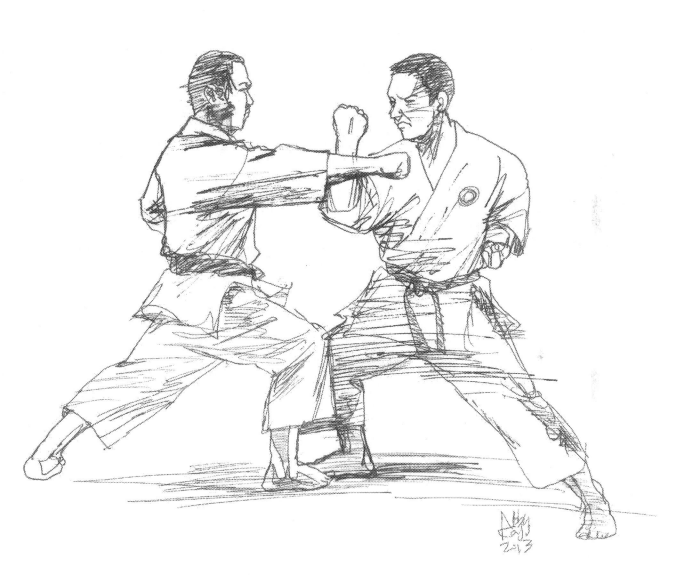

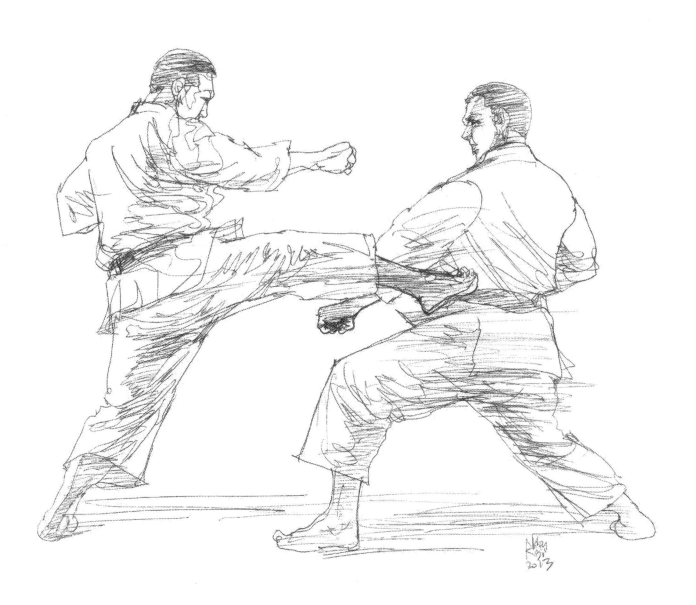

214

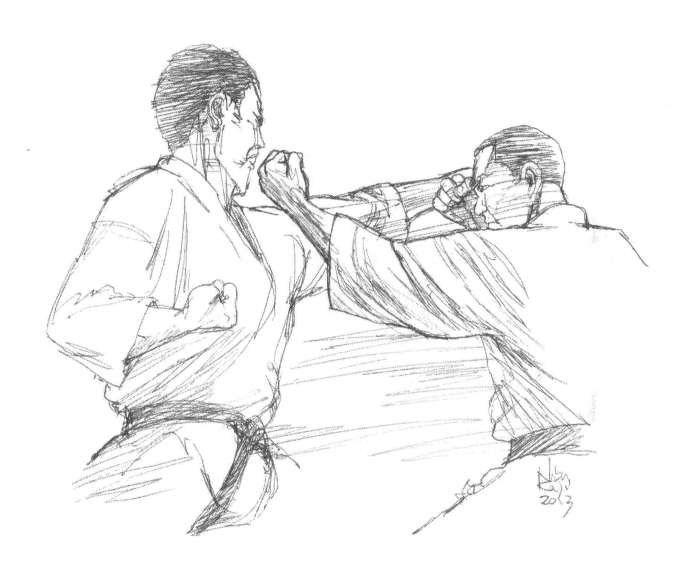

215

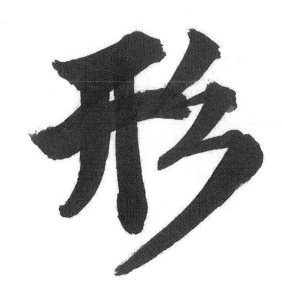

Kata

Heian Shodan

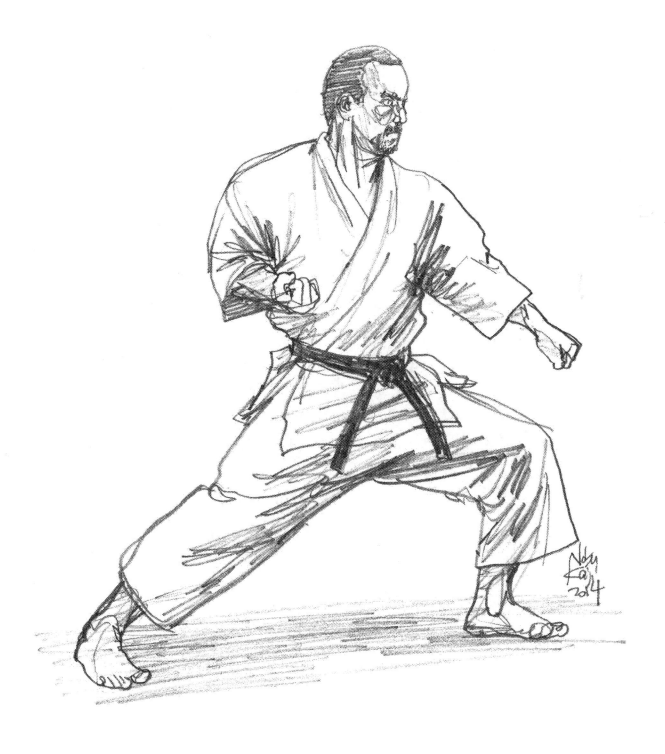

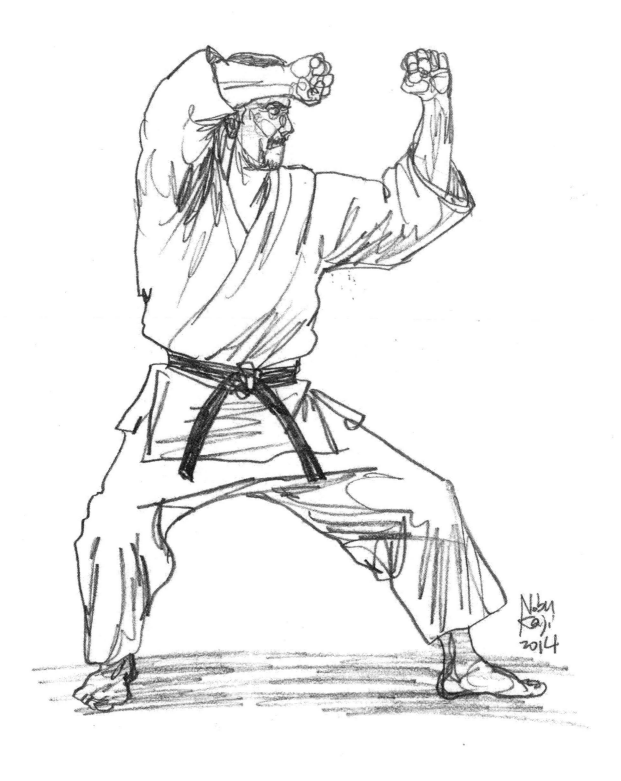

Heian Sandan

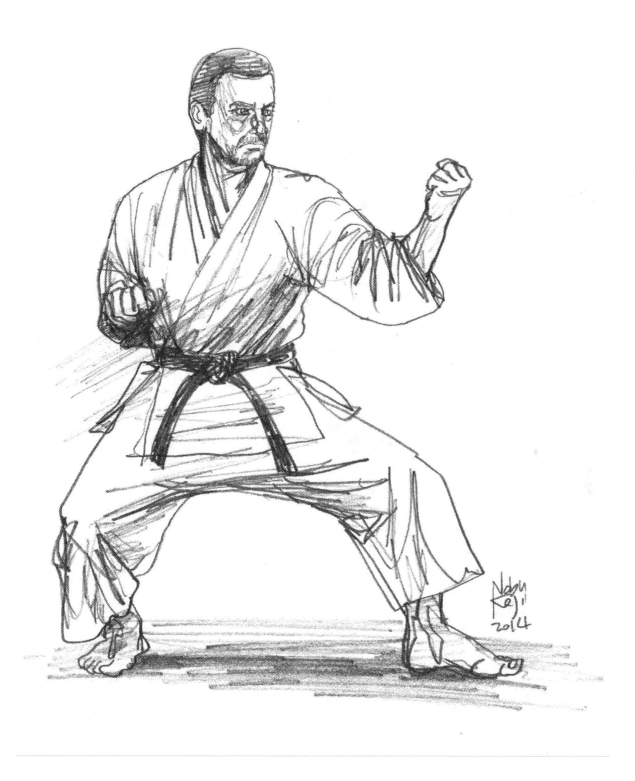

Heian Yondan

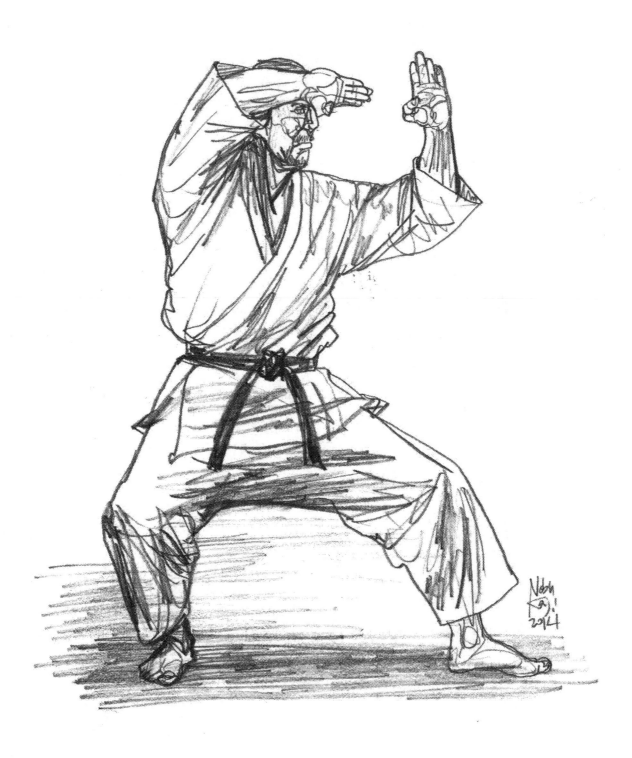

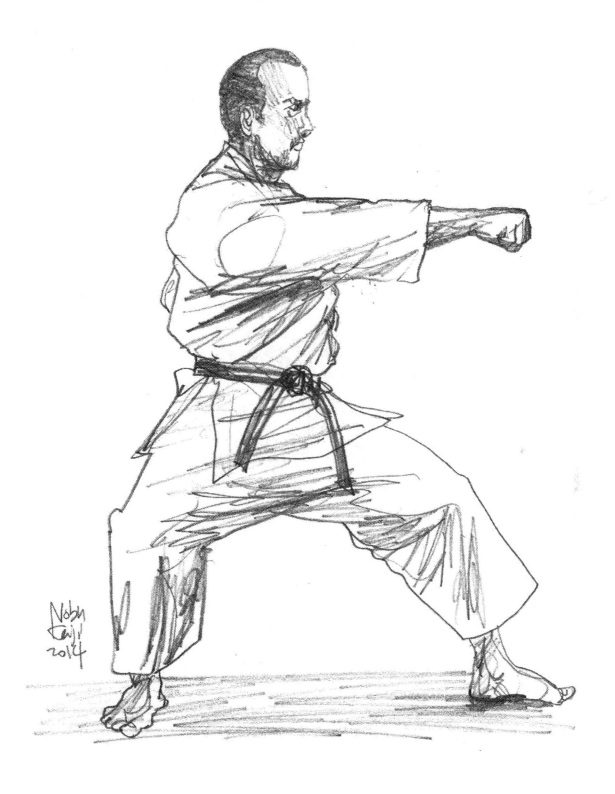

Tekki Shodan

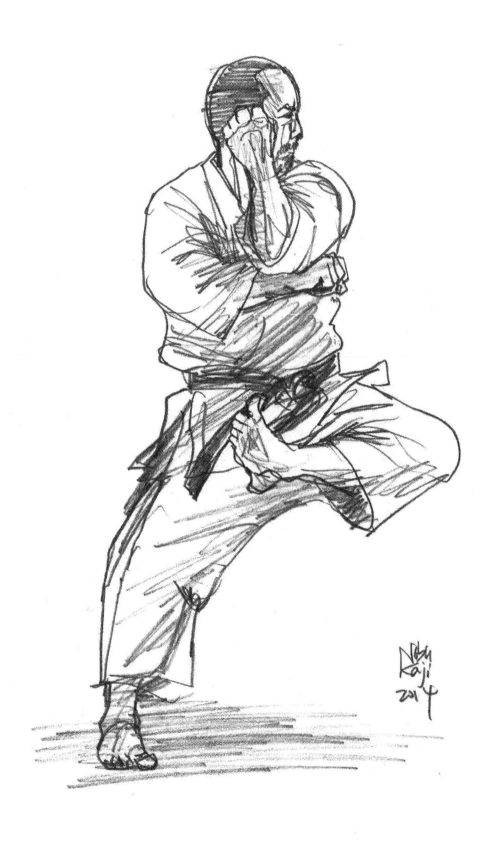

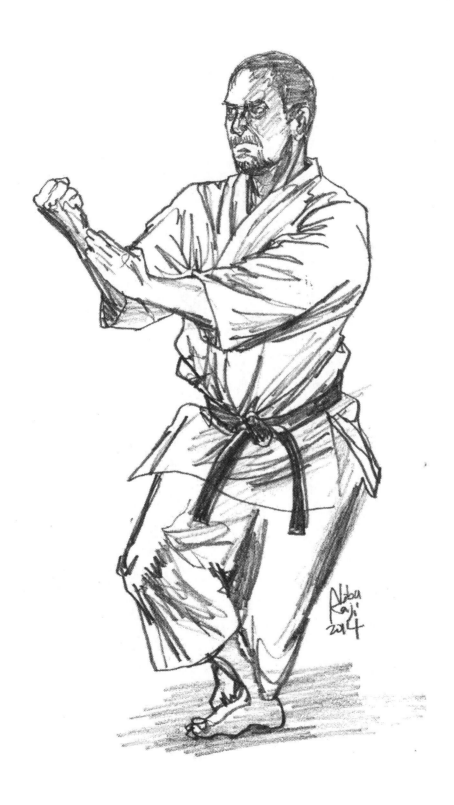

Jion

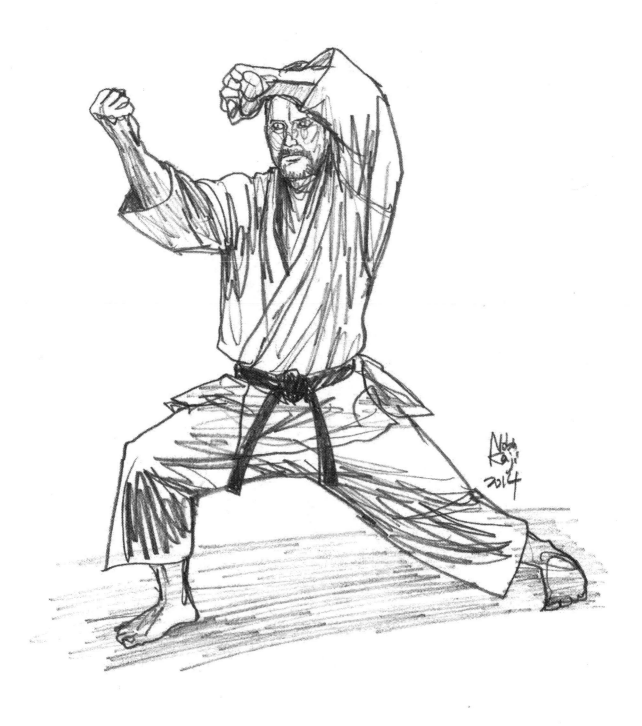

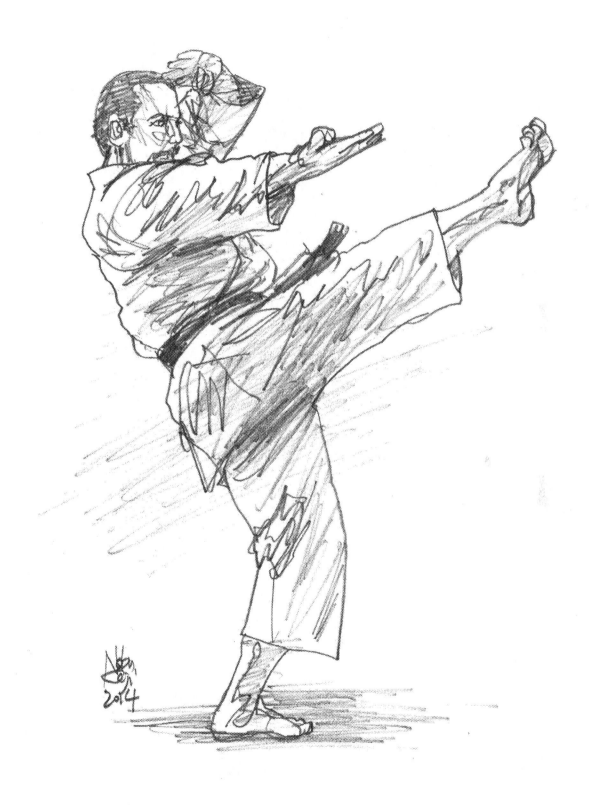

Hangetsu

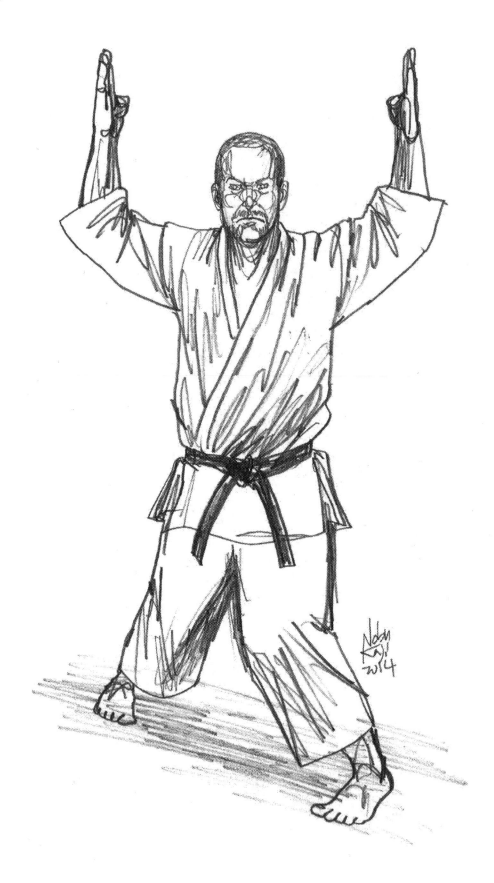

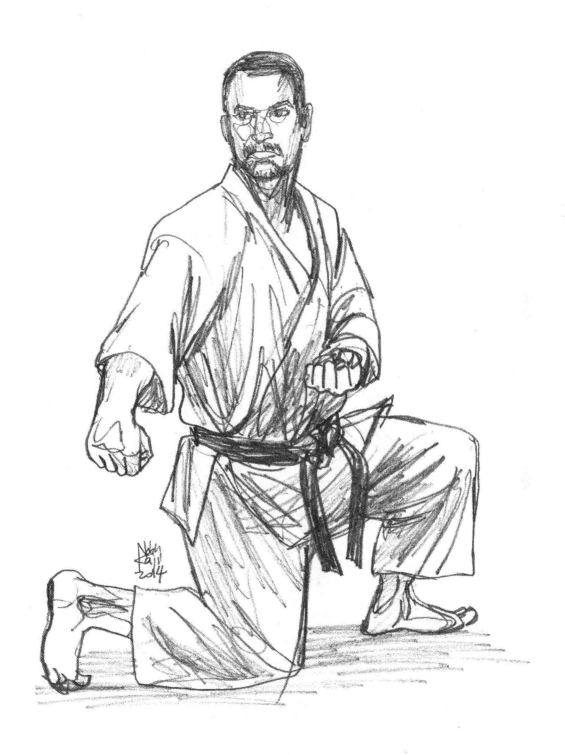

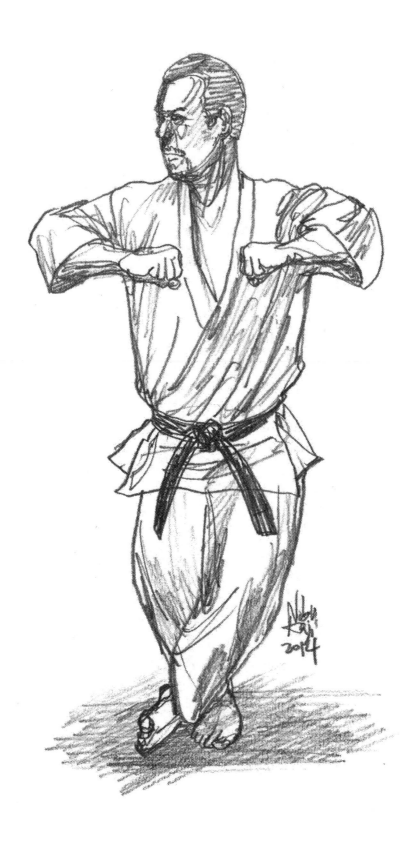

Bassai Sho

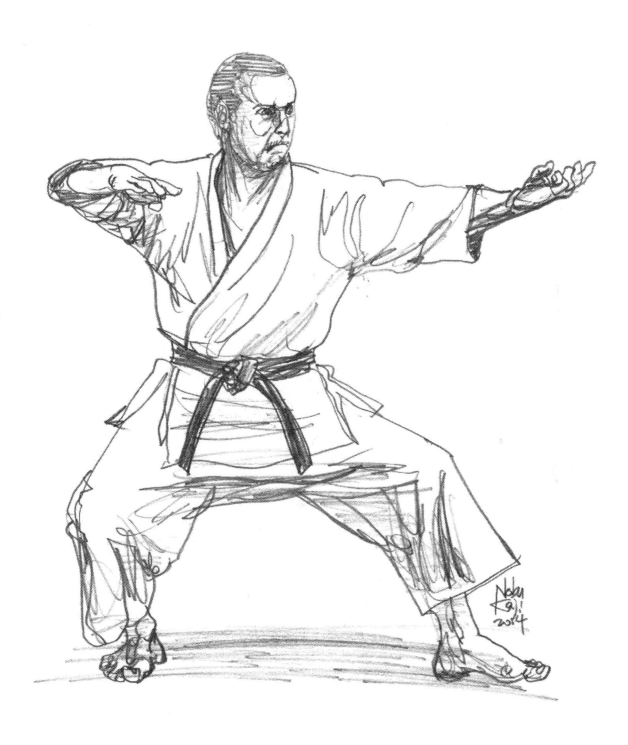

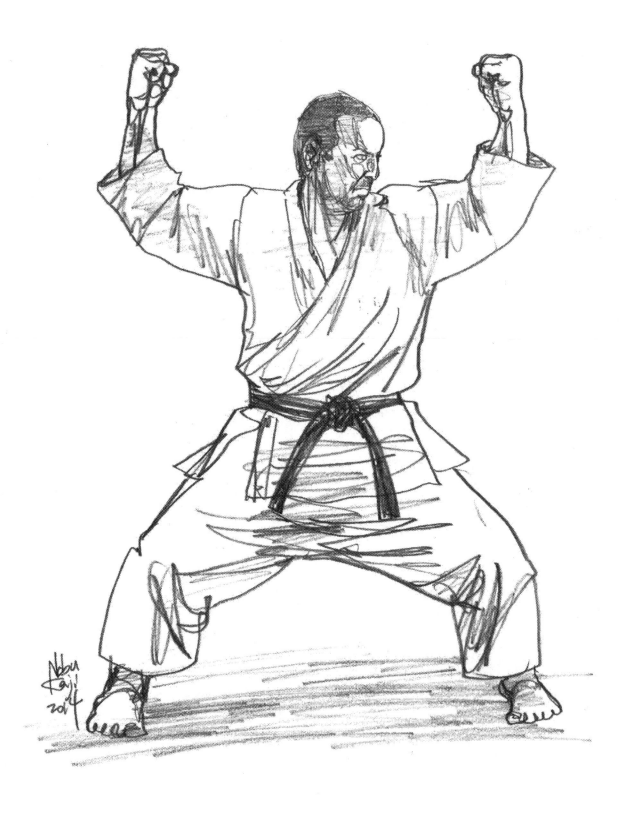

Kanku Sho

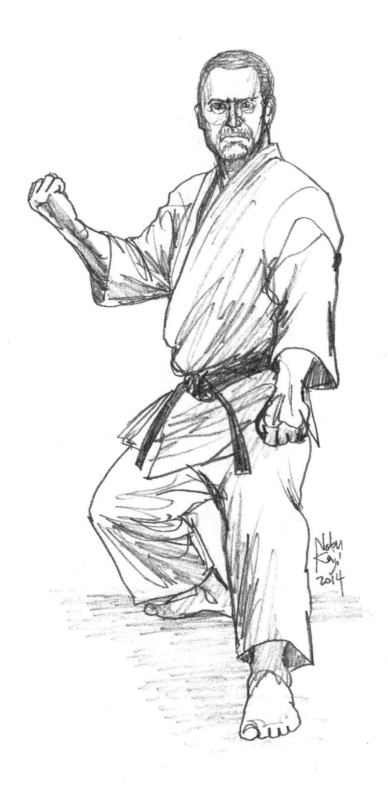

Chinte

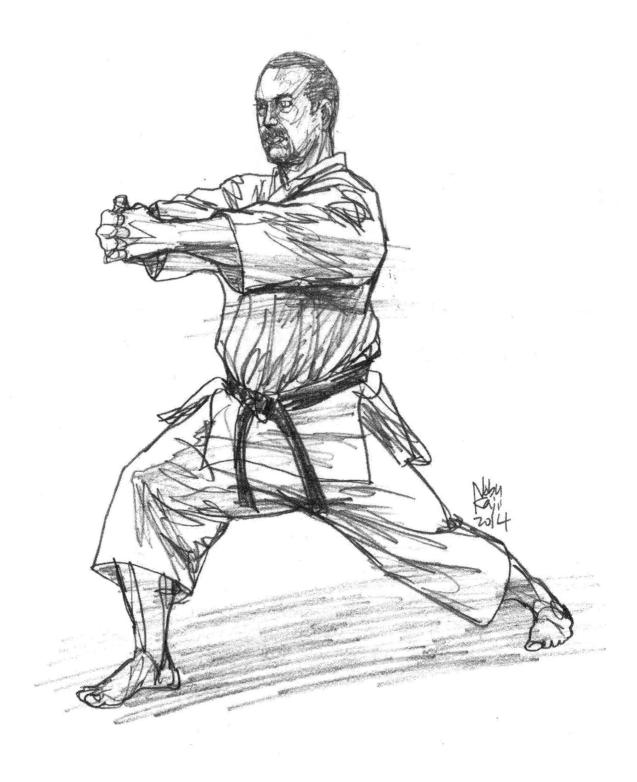

Jiin

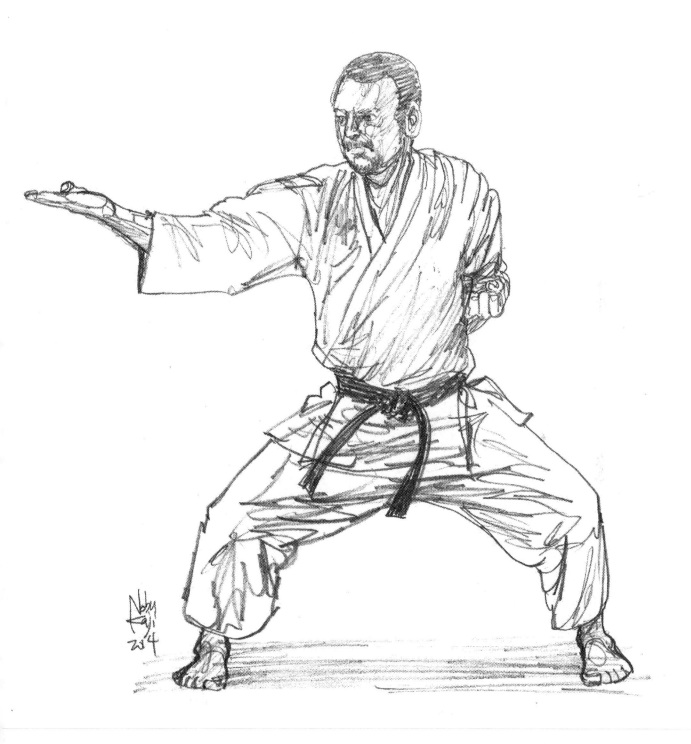

Tekki Sandan

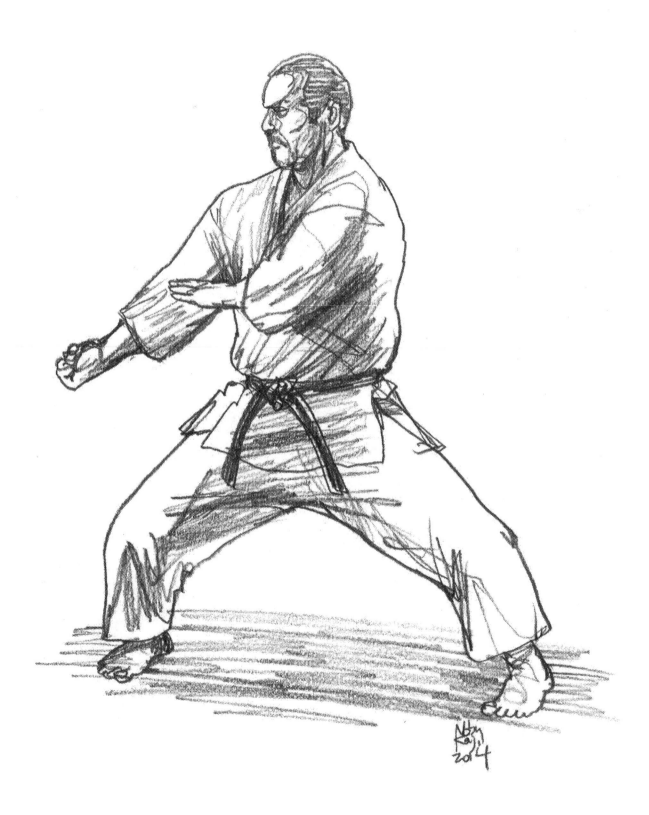

Gankaku

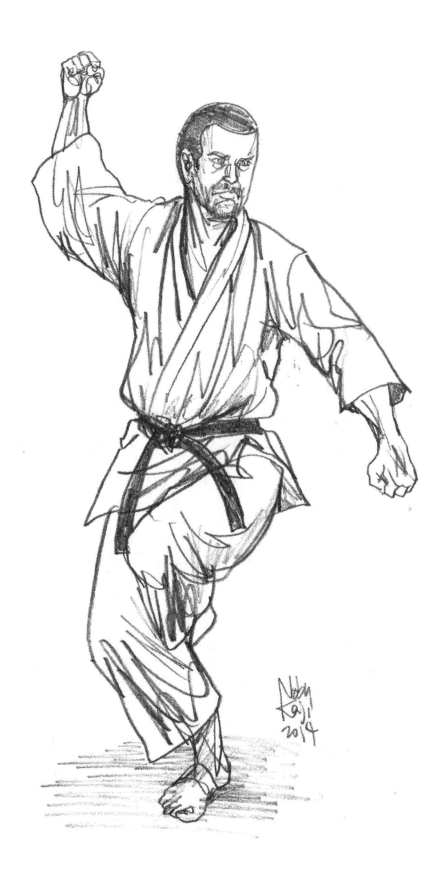

Sochin

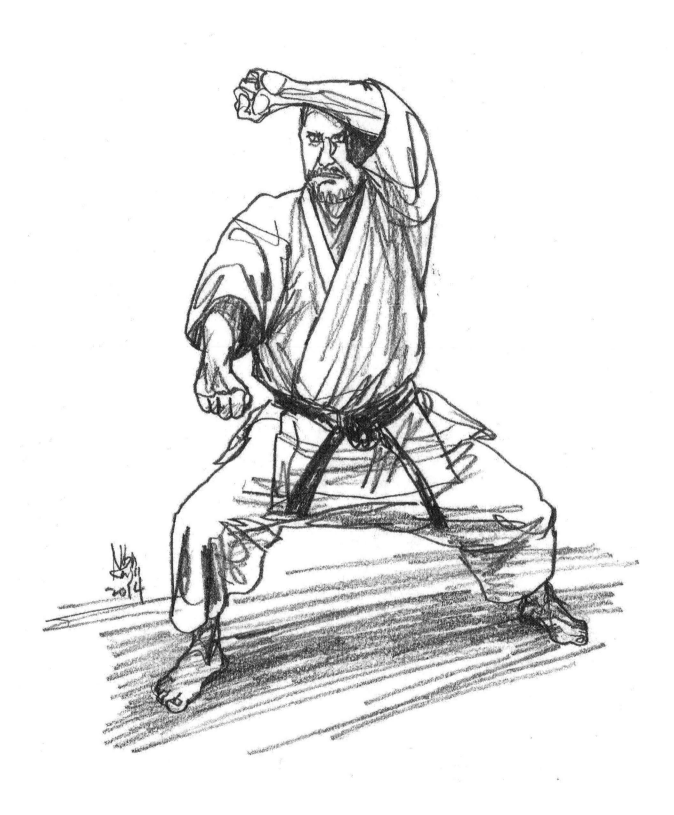

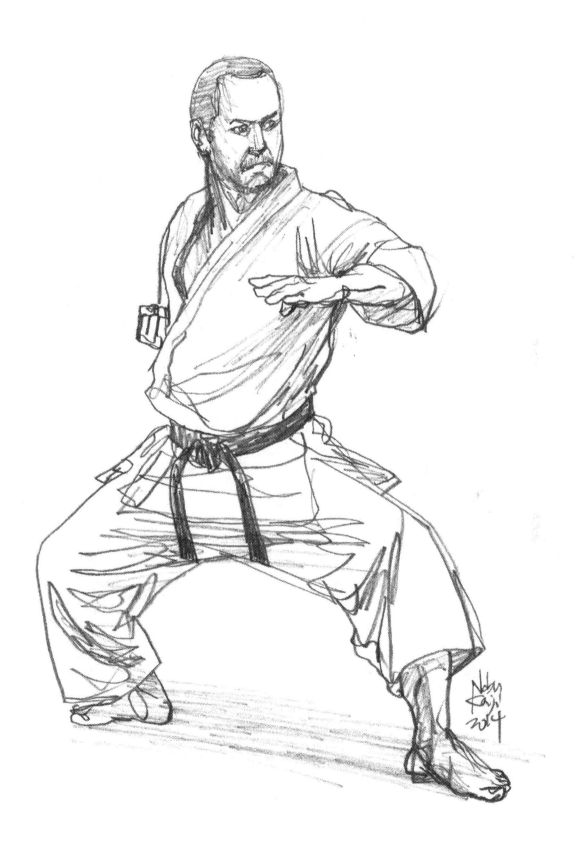

Meikyo

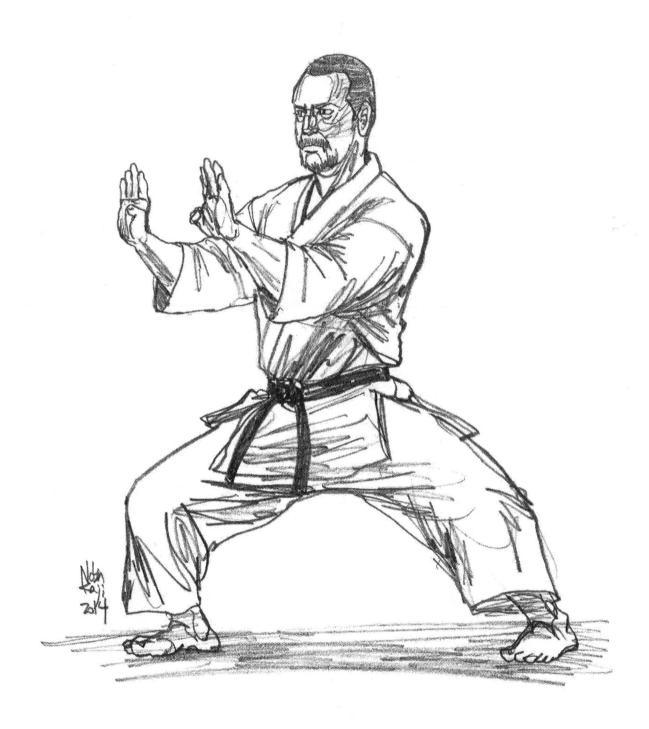

Wankan

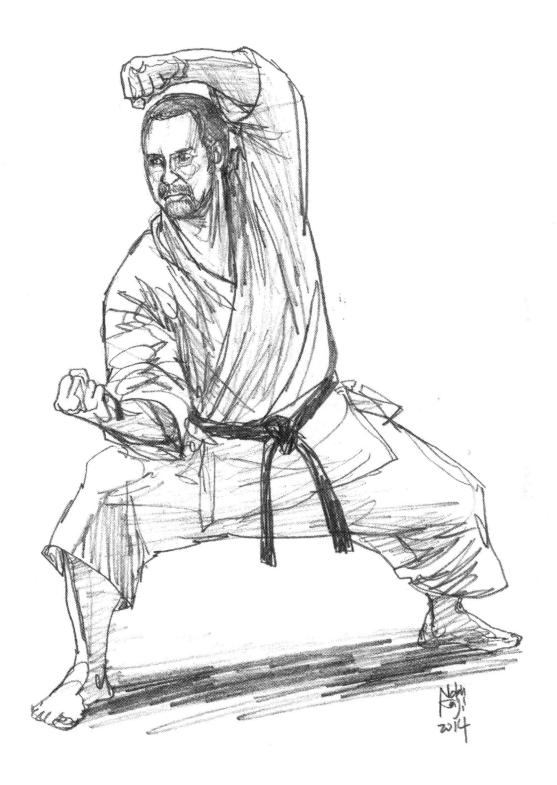

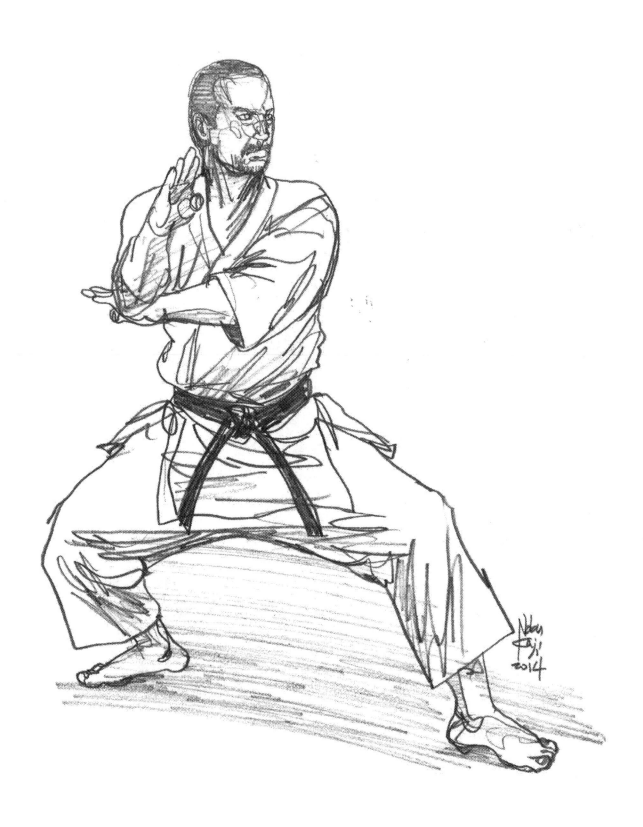

Goju Shi Ho Dai

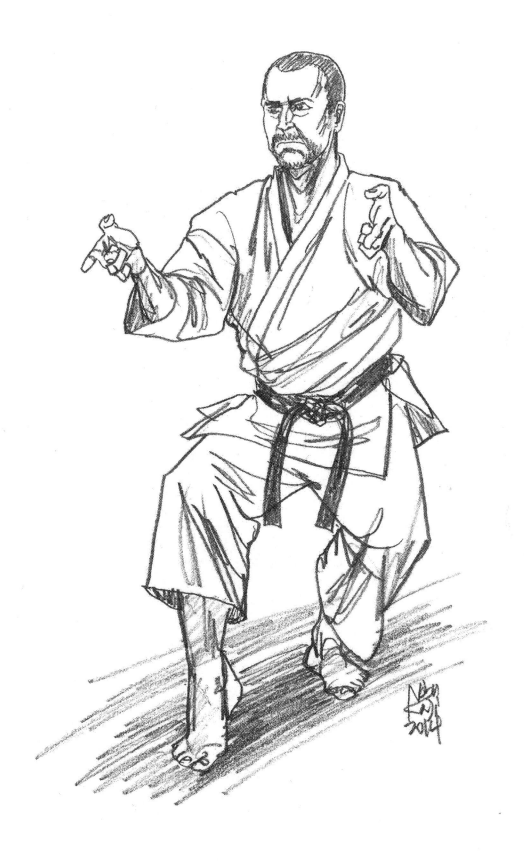

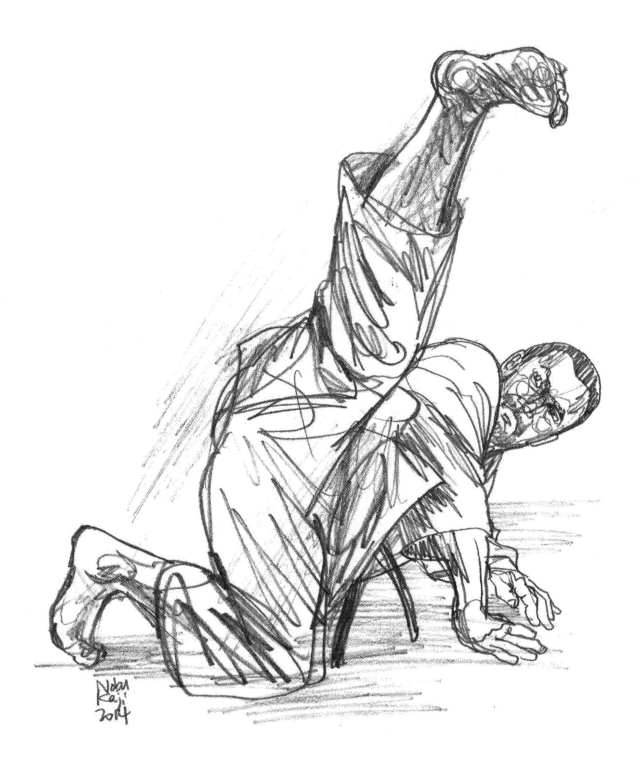

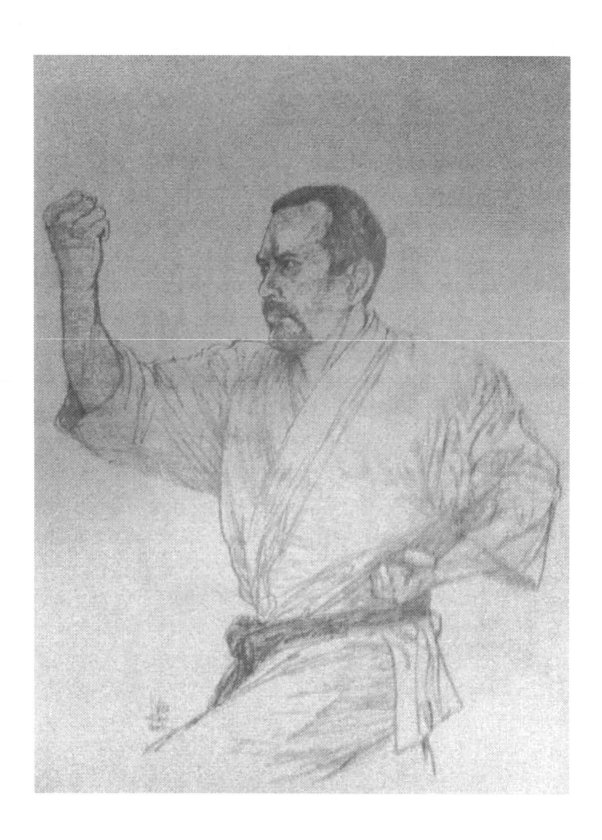

About the Author

(Luis) Bernardo Mercado has studied Shotokan Karate since 1981. While enrolled in the engineering program at San Francisco State University, he began training with sensei Mayer Parry, who was a direct student of kancho Hirokazu Kanazawa.

In 1983, Bernardo started training with sensei Leroy Rodrigues, who is founder and chief instructor of the Shinkyu Shotokan Karate dojo, at the South San Francisco Parks and Recreation Department.

Sensei Leroy Rodrigues awarded Bernardo a first degree black belt in Shotokan and Shorinji Ryu karate-do in 1986. Bernardo taught at the Shinkyu Shotokan Karate dojo in Orange Park for 20 years.

Upon moving to Fremont California in 1997, Bernardo continued studying martial arts with sensei Al McGaughey at the Pine Waves Karate Academy. In 2009, he partnered with sensei McGaughey and sensei Harry Imamura to founded the Fremont Shotokan Karate dojo, where all three currently teach and train.

Sensei Leroy Rodrigues awarded Bernardo a sixth degree black belt in Shotokan in 2007.

Concurrent with studying, training, teaching and competing in karate, in 1992 sensei Mercado partnered with his younger brother Ernesto and founded Core Power Services, Inc., where they both work with a great team of field engineers and office staff.

Mr. Mercado has contributed to two other martial arts books: *Classic Kata of Shorinji Ryu: Okinawan Karate Forms of Richard 'Biggie' Kim* by Leroy Rodrigues, and *Karate Everyone, 2nd Edition* by Steve McCann.

Mr. Mercado is also author of *Critical Thinking 101: Key Concepts for the American Voter,* a book with ideas and information designed to stimulate intellectual honesty, positive attitude, and an ethical lifestyle reflecting the way of martial arts.

Oss!

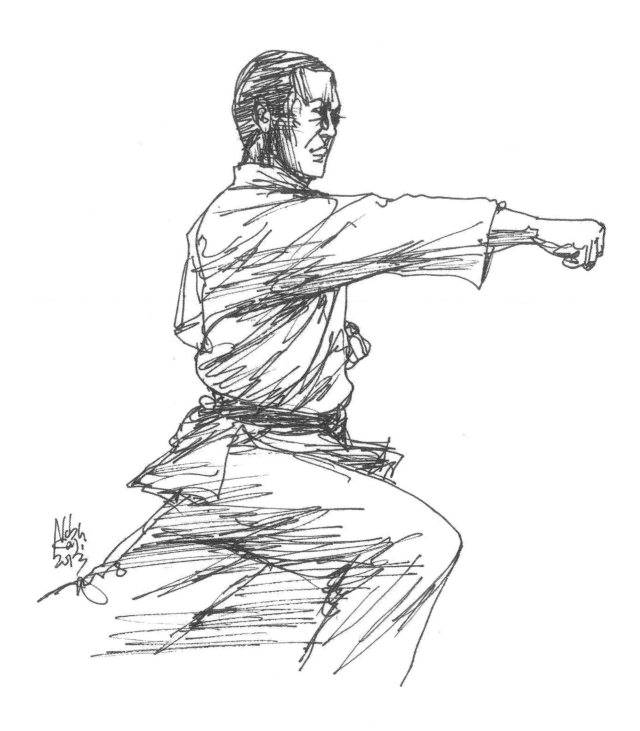